D0261994

YOUR GOOD HEALTH!

YOUR GOOD HEALTH!

The Medicinal Benefits of Wine Drinking

E. Maury

Translated by Della Couling

Souvenir Press

First published in France by
Éditions Artulen, Paris

First British Edition published 1992 by
Souvenir Press Ltd., 43 Great Russell Street, London WC1B 3PA
and simultaneously in Canada

ISBN 0 285 63096 2

Typeset by Rowland Phototypesetting Ltd., Bury St Edmunds, Suffolk
Printed in Great Britain by Mackays of Chatham PLC, Chatham, Kent

CONTENTS

Part Two
WINE AND THE FUNCTIONS

PREFACE

Throughout the world, whatever the customs and ethical or religious beliefs, we humans always seem to have needed to use stimulants to help us cope with psychological pressures of one sort or another, and particularly with pressures in our emotional lives.

For centuries, depending on climate and latitude, people have sought comfort from the effects of coffee, tea, tobacco or opium; but in the 1990s, natural mood elevators no longer seem adequate to satisfy this need, so that we are now turning to synthetic analeptics, or boosters, and more and more to sophisticated drugs that make fortunes for their creators. The consequences are obvious today.

However, in regions blessed with balmier skies and a more discerning culture, people turned to the cultivation of the vine and, for centuries, have been able to find in its product the satisfaction of their needs.

Sociologists and moral philosophers are agreed that any usage or practice which does not meet a need or fulfil a specific function soon declines and falls into neglect; but for thousands of years, in the Latin countries, wine has continued to be an integral part of daily life and habits.

This custom, rooted in tradition and wisdom, was respected until recent decades, which then witnessed the launching of a propaganda campaign aimed at discrediting the fermented juice of the grape, making it a scapegoat for every imaginable sin.

Under the banner of anti-alcoholism, laudable in itself in view of the evidence for alcohol abuse, and in particular aggravated by the dubious quality of liquids offered under the name of wine, which have nothing in common with a quality vintage, some well-intentioned worthies have unfortunately included wine among the substances whose consumption has been shown to have a damaging effect on the human body.

However, statistics have proved that alcohol abuse is far greater in those regions of France that are not wine-growing and which are therefore not habitual wine drinking communities.

If we really wished, in all honesty, to conduct a campaign against alcoholism, why not start by banning, by official control of medicinal products, the use of certain cough syrups intended for children, some even for infants, which have an alcoholic content approaching that of *digestifs* like cognac or calvados: this practice is promoting, in all good faith, a sort of precocious alcoholism.

If you really think about it, what has been the consequence of this anti-wine campaign, waged on behalf of public health? The results are only too obvious today.

The individual, badly informed and above all badly advised, deprived of his need for tranquillisers and relaxants, has instinctively turned to new sources that dispense oblivion and create euphoria. He seeks them now, and has done since adolescence, in drugs that become progressively 'harder', the craving for which leads to a steady increase in criminal activity and mental breakdown. The parallel increase in the number of drug addicts and the social and health consequences of this new epidemic should therefore come as no surprise.

While still on the same subject, we should remember that, during the Prohibition, instituted in the United States at the end of the First World War on the misguided initiative of water-drinking leagues, there had never been so many cases of drunkenness, caused by the illicit manufacture of alcohol of dubious origin. Thank heavens, more reasonable spirits realised the harmfulness of this 'aquatic' movement, and today American wine production is flourishing.

Until now, those of us in the old countries of Europe have been spared such excesses, but can one compare wine, a natural product created by the genius of man and solely intended for man, to an alcoholic substitute which is by definition toxic?

In a previous book* I looked at the fermented product of the vine from the angle of the most common illnesses, showing how, when such illnesses occur, wine can be used as a medicinal supplement.

In the following pages I shall be discussing the physiological and psychological effects of wine on the main functions of the body, and since this book is written under the aegis of Hippocrates, I shall try, in conclusion, to correlate the four temperaments described by the father of medicine with their opposite numbers in the world of wine.

* *Wine is the Best Medicine*, Souvenir Press, 1976.

PART ONE
A MEDICAL APPROACH TO WINE

'The vine, and wine, are great mysteries. Alone in the vegetable kingdom, the vine makes intelligible to us the true flavour of the earth.
What fidelity in the translation . . .
It holds, pressed from the grape, the secrets of the soil.'

COLETTE

CHAPTER 1

FROM VINE TO VAT

For thousands of years *Homo sapiens* has required the produce of the earth to supply him not only with the elements essential to his survival, but also with those which, if need be, will help him to combat illness. The cultivation of the fertile soil combined with an improved knowledge of plants has allowed him to fulfil this double aim.

These time-honoured needs can be rediscovered in modern terms, by following a well-balanced diet and by an increasing reliance on the medicinal properties of certain herbs. With her abundance of plants, Nature provides remedies for all our bodily ailments, whatever they may be. Our modern chemists, who have become aware of these herbal properties, try in the secrecy of their laboratories to reconstitute the formula artificially. But their synthetic products often turn out to be more harmful to the users than the symptoms they are meant to be treating. Let us leave these scientists to their test-tubes, and stick to those medicinal agents which are closer to their natural origin, and so better adapted to human kind.

If the vine belongs unequivocally to the realm of plant biology, then we can in all good faith assume that the same applies to its final product that we owe to the work of vine-growers: the fermented juice of the vine. After all, does not the grape cure itself belong to phytotherapy, or herbal medicine?

Before discussing the effect of wine on the main organic functions and to give us a clearer understanding of how it works, let us first reconsider the constituent parts of this climbing and trailing shrub of the family Vitaceae.

Leaves and Pips

The vine (*Vitis vinifera*) consists of branches, palmate leaves, clusters of self-pollinating flowers and, at maturity, fruits, which are the grape clusters. In their turn, these are made up of two parts: a woody section—the stalk—and the berries, composed of skin, pips and pulp, the crushing of which produces the juice or must.

The aim of this deliberately brief description is to bring out the role which this shrub can play in our physical and mental health, whenever we feel a need for it.

I shall not dwell on the sartorial use that has been made of the leaf, except to recall that, since the earthly Paradise was lost by our first ancestors, who were also the first nudists, this part of the vine has merely been used aesthetically by painters and sculptors who feared that their works might offend innocent eyes. Fortunately, in our day, more relaxed moral attitudes have helped to make this use of the leaf totally obsolete. The vine leaf today has other uses.

There was a time when doctors used the properties of red vine leaves as a remedy for uterine haemorrhages. This action on the blood came from their richness in anthocyanic pigments. A present-day phytotherapist, Henri Leclerc, likes to mix them in an infusion with fumitory and marjoram to alleviate the problems of women who have reached or passed a certain age.

In the same way, other doctors have utilised the healing properties of these vine leaves in the form of a liquid alcoholic extract in the treatment of haemorrhoids and phlebitis. It is interesting to point out, right at the beginning of this book, the beneficial influence of the vine on blood circulation. Later on we shall be returning to this question. As for the pips, because of their rich tannin content they were formerly recommended as an astringent remedy for treating the symptoms of tuberculosis, when doctors had to deal with haemorrhagic complications.

The Fruit

This is the part of the vine which, from the medicinal point of view, has the widest range of applications.

In its fresh state, the pulp of the grape contains 80 per cent water and 20 per cent sugar in the form of glucose, mannite, laevulose and dulcite. The proportion of these glucidic components depends on the quality and amount of sunshine the fruit receives throughout the time when it is ripening. This factor explains why the southern regions produce grapes richer in sugar and consequently wines with a higher degree of alcohol.

In addition to these basic components, the juice of the grape is rich in proteins drawn from the roots and leaves, as well as in mineral salts.

The latter include calcium, magnesium, potassium, sodium, silica, sulphur, phosphorus and chloride. Also important are organic acids which come from the roots and leaves, and trace elements and vitamins. Most of the latter belong to the B complex. Grape juice also contains elements related to vitamin P.

All these components are also found in wine, but at that stage in the transformation of grape juice, their activity increases thanks to the fermentation process undergone by the must.

As for the skin of the fruit, it plays a mechanical role by providing roughage. It helps to stimulate the flow of digestive juices and aids bowel function.

The Grape Cure

The different properties of these natural elements mean that together they provide an effective medicinal action—an action increased, however, after fermentation.

In current practice, the grape cure consists in eating the fruit as it is, in its solid form, or drinking its juice after it has been pressed. This form of therapy demands on average the daily consumption of two to three kilos of fresh grapes. It has a beneficial effect on health by helping to strengthen the body's resistance to bacterial or viral attacks, and it also helps to combat fatigue during convalescence. Diuretic and purgative through its action on the kidneys and liver, it plays a part in cleansing organs clogged up by organic waste. Furthermore, its alkalising power modifies a tendency to acidification of the humoral areas, important in treating arthritis cases. Finally, this cure offers the main nutritive elements which are essential for healthy function of the whole body.

It is therefore prescribed as a medicinal supplement to other treatments, in cases of skin complaints, rheumatic symptoms and hypertension. It is also recommended for those suffering from overweight, habitual constipation and flatulence.

I mention these medicinal effects of fresh grape juice in order to highlight the importance of its various components in phytotherapeutic treatment. These become even more apparent following the fermentation process, when the juice of the grape has acquired new credentials and, medically speaking, can then be considered from a different point of view.

CHAPTER 2

FROM OSIRIS TO PASTEUR . . . AND BEYOND

Before looking at the medicinal uses of wine down the centuries, I should like to make a point of a linguistic nature, since I want to avoid any possible confusion or misunderstanding about what I mean. If we are to appreciate how wine can benefit our health it is quite important to be precise in our use of words, especially in relation to problems of illness or malfunction.

A Definition

The product of the vine is not a *medicine* to be prescribed as a substitute for those which the sick person may be advised to take in allopathic or orthodox treatment. The fermented juice of the vine must be considered as a 'supplement', taken by the patient merely as a *remedy*.

There is a different between these two terms. They both define agents which work together in the treatment of illness and the restoration of health. By *medicine* I mean any substance, simple or compound, administered internally or externally as an 'aid to health'; by *remedy*, all the other elements likely to be given for a therapeutic purpose, for the greater good of the patient.

Having made clear this distinction, and in the spirit of this book, we shall consider wine as a 'supplementary remedy', meaning by this everything that can bring about a beneficial change in the physiological functioning of any limb or organ, and their return to full health, whether such means are hygienic, pharmaceutical, physiotherapeutic, surgical or even dietary.

By its nature, the vine belongs to the vegetable world, so its end-product, wine, can be classed as a phytotherapeutic, and therefore natural, agent. This opinion is shared by a good number of practitioners. At the time of the Agricultural Congress in France in 1939, Doctor Cuvier, with the support of Professor Perrot of the Faculty of Pharmacy in Paris, classified *Vitis vinifera* among the number of medicinal plants. I have given reasons for this in the preceding chapter.

These experts merely endorsed the opinion of those doctors who, from time immemorial, have accepted, if not encouraged, the use of wine as a medicinal aid. A brief look back into history, with a detour into mythology, will serve to confirm the main thesis of this book.

The Ancient World

The earliest references to the medicinal virtues attributed to the juice of the vine seem to date from around five thousand years ago. In those distant times, in Ancient Egypt, Osiris, god of vegetation, son of Heaven and Earth, brother and husband of Isis, was the first to cultivate the vine. In recognition of this happy stroke of genius, he was called 'Master of the Flowering Vine'. A myth that we cannot ignore, since it concerns wine, told of this god being reborn from his own ashes. So he triumphed over Death, just as every year the grape is reborn from a vinestock that during the winter looks quite dead. By analogy, we could liken this imagery to that of convalescence after illness.

Thousands of years later Noah, the biblical patriarch whose name is always coupled with wine, repeated in his turn the creative action of the Egyptian god. After the retreat of the muddy waters left by the Flood, he planted the vine on soil which had once more become fertile, thereby marking the dawn of a new era for humanity. Wine was its symbol. And a little later Moses, leading his people towards the Promised Land, sent messengers, among them Caleb and Joshua, to explore its agricultural potential. They returned from the land of Canaan with a cluster of grapes as proof of its fruitfulness. Subsequently wine and its benefits were cited more than 450 times in the Bible, and the Babylonian Talmud considered it the most effective of medicines.

Leaving the eastern shores of the Mediterranean, we reach the land of Greece, cradle of our western civilisation. There, instead of Osiris, we find Dionysos, son of Zeus and Semele. This mythical character was known throughout the Hellenic world as the god of sap and was later consecrated god of the vine. His whole story is shot through with symbols relating to wine. From his birth he was entrusted to the care of the nymphs of Mount Nysa, and he grew up in the shade of a grotto, like the juice of the vine which ferments and matures in the secrecy of the vault. Having pressed the juice of the grape, the young god gave the fermented wine to his nurses to sample, and the outcome of this first 'wine-tasting' session persuaded him that mankind should share in the joys of his discovery.

It was not long before these myths became a reality—from the very start of the historical period, when the medicinal properties of wine were officially recognised. From that time men replaced the gods.

The fermented juice of the vine made its entry into the field of therapeutics with Hippocrates. Grandson of a king, born in the first year of the 83rd Olympiad at the Temple of Asclepius of Cos, he was raised and initiated in the medical tradition by priests serving the cult of Asclepius. Creator of the Humoral Doctrine, which will be discussed again in the last part of this book when we consider its relationship with wine, he reminds us in his *Aphorisms* that 'wine is a thing marvellously suited to man if, in health as in sickness, it is administered appropriately and in just measure in accordance with the individual constitution.' Applying these principles, he advises the use of white wine in cases of dropsy.* What is more, he claims that this beverage has a beneficial effect on a sluggish stomach, as it revives the appetite, nourishes and fortifies the body. Then moving on to wider themes, he praises the stamina of wine and its ability to make people like gods.

Rich in his teaching, he founded the Hippocratic School, which blamed melancholy or the 'Sad Humour' for causing any number of illnesses. Hence, the treatment for this mental state, which affects the body in various ways, tended towards a quest for gaiety which helped to 'dilate the passages of the spleen'. This psychosomatic view of illness has recently been regaining favour. Even in those far-off times, however, the use of wine for medicinal purposes was thought likely to restore 'good humours', terms which, according to their Hippocratic meaning, correspond to each of the four organic fluids circulating in the human body: bile, black bile, phlegm and blood. We should add that these 'humours' the Greek doctor is talking about are still present in any living organism; they merely go under different names. Although blood is still known by the name it had then, nowadays the other fluids are described respectively as lymph and interstitial fluid.

Before leaving ancient Greece and the shores of the Ionian Sea, it is worth recalling the properties attributed at the time to the wines of Cernya in Achaea, which were reputed to make barren women fertile. On the other

* A condition in which fluid accumulates in the body's membranes and connective tissues.

hand, those not wishing to continue with their pregnancy were advised to drink the wine of Troezen, cultivated in Argolis, the city of the tragic love that broke Phaedra's heart. Perhaps these candidates for abortion followed the advice of Galen of Pergamum, the famous doctor who recommended getting drunk at least once a month.

In ancient Rome, Bacchus replaced Dionysos. The Dionysiac became the Bacchanalia. Here too, the product of the vine lost none of its therapeutic qualities. Several authors bear witness to this.

Pliny the Elder, the naturalist who fell victim to his own professional curiosity at Pompeii at the time of the eruption of Vesuvius in AD79, recalled in his *Natural History* the medicinal uses of the vine shoot, its leaves and pips. He adds this sentence which agrees with Hippocratic teaching and confirms the action of the fermented juice of the vine: 'wine in itself is a remedy; it nourishes the blood of man, it delights the stomach and soothes care and affliction.'

In his turn, Celsus, a physician of the time of Augustus, endorsed Galen's ideas regarding the beneficial influence of wine on health. He recommends wine to accompany diets which he classifies as 'heating', meaning foods which should be eaten by people who are anaemic.

There is every indication that the Romans of the period assiduously followed this good advice, if we look at the account Petronius has left us of the famous banquet given by Trimalchio, who said to his guests: 'Wine lives longer than man; so let us drink like sponges, for wine is life.'

The Middle Ages

After the collapse of the Roman Empire in the West

following the invasion of the barbarians from the East, the tradition of wine-making, like the phoenix reborn from its ashes, was revived and maintained in the obscurity of monastic cellars. Throughout centuries of turmoil, the vine continued to thrive, especially in the precincts of the monasteries, among the most renowned of these being Cluny and Citeaux in Burgundy, the land of good wine. Saint Benedict of Aniane, to whose order the monastery of Cluny belonged, aware of the digestive virtues of the juice of the vine, recommended its consumption during monastic meals, to the amount of one 'hemin' (about a quarter of a litre), so that the monks might remain always *digesti et alacres*, in other words, in top form.

The above advice reminds us that throughout the ages the juice of the vine has always been regarded as having a spiritual quality. It is an indication of the symbolism that surrounded this beverage in medieval times. The vinestock which renewed its greenery every spring symbolised the Resurrection and the wine was likened to the blood of Christ who nurtured the human spirit throughout his time on earth.

Faithful to the doctrine that preaches the union of things spiritual and temporal, the alchemists of the time tried to establish a link between the vine which, of all plants, is best suited to our temperament, and mankind who is privileged to enjoy its quintessence.

In Hermetic Medicine,* of which the Swiss physician and alchemist Paracelsus (*c.*1490–1541) was one of the best known advocates, wine was considered a panacea capable of curing all ills. In Paracelsus' opinion, the fermented juice of the vine not only warms the 'humid and cold' temperament, but also helps to refresh one that

* Named after Hermes Trismegistus, the third-century author of Neoplatonic writings on mysticism and alchemy.

is 'dry and hot', a theory akin to the Hippocratic concept of illness.

In spite of this old-fashioned terminology, these images nevertheless express a physiological truth. Instead of dismissing this approach to the invalid as obsolete, I shall attempt to prove, in the course of this book, that the medicinal choice of a particular wine corresponds, by its action on the main functions of the body, to a clinical reality and a therapeutic purpose.

Espousing wholeheartedly the ideas of the Hermetic practitioners, the followers of the Doctrine of Signatures* regarded white wine as drinkable gold, *aurum potabile*, reflecting the sun which penetrates the grape to suffuse it with its radiance, while red wine corresponds to the blood, having its colour and heat.

Before leaving the Middle Ages, we must mention the medical school at Salerno, south of Naples, which recommended the use of wine, claiming that it would bestow vigour and rejuvenate the aged. However, the masters of this school added to their counsels a final word of advice regarding moderation: 'Drink little but well.'

The Renaissance

At this time a vaster knowledge of the world opened up and this only served to confirm the medicinal virtues of wine. Its main advocate and propagandist was none other than the French writer Françqis Rabelais (*c.*1494–1553), who was a respected doctor of medicine at the School of Montpellier; he proclaimed to all and sundry: 'The juice of the vine clears the mind and the under-

* A signature was a distinctive mark, or a peculiarity of shape or colouring, which was thought to indicate the qualities for medicinal purposes of a plant or other natural object.

standing, banishes sadness, imparts gladness and jollity.'

His near contemporary, Michel de Montaigne (1533–1592), moralist and wine-grower, dealt with his bladder stones by taking, for preference, a little dry white wine.

Not only that, whenever he went travelling around Europe, in quest of culture and learning, he never failed to stop at the shores of Lake Geneva to undergo a cure based on the Villeneuve *petit cru* which possesses acknowledged diuretic properties. This wine-loving philosopher voiced his allegiance to the principles of the above-mentioned Salerno school, when he wrote these lines in his *Essays*: 'I have heard Sylvius, that excellent physician from Paris, say that, to preserve the powers of the stomach and prevent them from becoming sluggish, it is a good idea, once a month, to wake them up by drinking too much wine and irritate them to stop them going to sleep.' This course of action was also followed by the Dutch humanist Erasmus (*c*.1466–1536), who relied on the virtues of the wine of Beaune to shake up his sluggish digestion. As for Ambroise Paré (1510–1590), surgeon to the French court, he applied poultices of red wine to wounds received by soldiers in battle. This treatment has been better understood since the discovery of the antibiotic properties of the Médoc wines.

The Universal Pharmacopœia, which appeared in 1677, contains a recipe for Samaritan's Balm. This preparation was based on a mixture of equal parts oil and red wine and was used for cleaning wounds. Taken internally, it helped cure catarrh and strengthen the nerves. This early type of medicinal wine was followed by a whole series of others, all based on grape juice, but containing macerations of medicinal plants such as digitalis (for *Vin de Trousseau*), scilla (for *Vin de la Charité*), colchicum, onion, even meat juices, peptones, citrate or ferrous tartrate.

Since the Age of Enlightenment

The nearer we come to the present day, so has wine, as its properties became better known, tended to occupy a more and more important place in medicinal prescriptions.

Leaving aside for a moment the Moliéresque treatments based on purges and blood-letting, Fagon, physician in ordinary to the Sun King Louis XIV, advised his illustrious patient, when he was suffering from an attack of gout, to replace the Burgundy which featured on the royal menu with a Champagne wine. As for Helvétius who gave his services to the Regent, the Duke of Orleans, out of a total of sixty prescriptions for his patient, in over twenty he recommended the use of wine for medicinal purposes. One of these prescriptions consisted of a certain tincture of tartar in a white wine base, a marvellous remedy, he maintained, for treating kidney and bladder ailments. It was this practitioner who declared that 'there is nothing wrong with wine taken in moderation, as it is useful and even necessary to facilitate digestion and fortify the stomach of the convalescent.'

This was also the opinion of the late eighteenth-century experimental chemist Antoine Francois Fourcroy: 'Wine,' he wrote, 'is an excellent remedy for those who do not habitually make use of it. It is a tonic, a stomachic, a corroborant [energising factor], a very powerful cordial.'

Since that time, many leading lights in the medical world have credited wine with medicinal virtues over and above its mere digestive benefits. Here we should note that, paradoxically, these arguments in favour of the fermented juice of the grape have often come from the Anglo-Saxon countries, although, as we know, under Cromwell wine-growing was actually forbidden in a misguided attempt to restore purity and righteousness.

By the 1780s, however, William Heberden was recommending those patients suffering from angina pectoris to take a glass of good claret at the onset of an attack. And his Scottish colleague, John Brown (1735–88), disdaining for once the whisky of his native land, advocated the red wines of Bordeaux to fight physical fatigue and psychological depression.

As for the German writer E.T.A. Hoffmann (1776–1822), he classed Chambertin as one of the 'poetic' wines while vaunting the merits of Champagne as a sovereign remedy for headache.

With the passing of the years, the medicinal use of wine has become more specific and more widespread. In 1822 the French physiologist Francçis Magendie (1783–1855) prescribed Bordeaux wine for cholera victims. And a little later, in 1886, during a fresh epidemic of this disease, Rambuteau had wine added to drinking water as a prophylactic. Other practitioners, such as Chomel, Sabrazes and Mercadier, had established the bactericidal power of Médoc on the typhoid bacillus.

Similarly, Gigon and the physiologist Charles Richet (1850–1935), winner of the 1913 Nobel Prize for Medicine, found that the Sauternes wines could destroy colon bacilli, a fact also established by the Viennese physician Pieck, who had shown that when polluted water was mixed with one third wine, it ceased to be toxic. Nor should we forget that in 1950 Professor Lancepleine attributed the bactericidal power of red wine to the fact that it contained the coloured pigments of the fruits. Above all, it was the important work of Professor Masquelier of Bordeaux and his colleagues, including Madame Jensen, that confirmed the antibiotic properties of red wines. These same researchers also discovered the beneficial effect on arteriosclerosis sufferers of including the Médoc vintages in their diet.

Finally, it would be impossible to end this historical

survey of uses of wine without mentioning the name of one of its most fervent supporters, Louis Pasteur, who extolled its cleansing properties when taken sensibly, in moderation.

CHAPTER 3
THE NOBILITY OF WINE

'If wine ceased to be produced, I believe that a vacuum would be left in the health and in the intelligence of our planet, a lack even more terrible than all the excesses for which it is blamed.'

The opinion expressed here by the French poet Charles Baudelaire (1821–67) is an exact reflection of the thinking behind this book: to show how the fermented juice of the vine, when used knowledgeably, can benefit us in mind and body.

Before going into detail about the use of wine as a universal remedy and giving some guidelines for treatment, I must first make a point that is really a matter of common sense. All living things, whether animal or vegetable, feel thirsty from time to time. When that happens, just a drink of pure water, mineralised or flavoured, will satisfy this natural craving. No one, surely, would think of offering a thirsty dog a saucer of Bordeaux, or of watering a dried-up vegetable patch with a generous sprinkling from a barrel of Muscadet. As the French writer J.-K. Huysmans (1848–1907) remarked, wine is a 'sacramental' substance, even if it is just an ordinary table wine—so long as it is a good one, of course.

Respect for Wine

For the Rev. Masquelier, who will be referred to several times in the course of this book, 'wine is more than a mere dilution of ethanol. It is the cellular content of the mature fruit, altered by fermentation. It occupies a very special place because of the number, variety and quality of its non-alcoholic constituents.'

As the natural outcome of the fermentation of grape juice, wine should not be treated merely as a way of replenishing lost body fluids or of washing down food. Its role is infinitely greater. The very act of sipping rather than gulping it helps to create the right balance in the body's functions. But this in turn helps to inspire the noblest human activities, which alone entitles wine to a certain respect and to be placed in the front rank of the earth's bounty, in the noble company of oil and bread.

Was it not Paul Claudel who said that 'wine is a teacher of taste and in training us to look inward, it is the liberator of the mind and the illuminator of the intelligence'? In its close union with the soul that feeds it, the vine absorbs essential ingredients. The sun's rays in their turn play their part in working what can only be described as an alchemy within the fruit itself. Extracted at last by the patient and unremitting toil of those who devote themselves to this task, the juice of the vine is thus enriched by a soil that takes on the character of its native wine-growing region and gives each vintage its unique quality. The vinestock absorbs it and the resultant juice, which is a synthesis of it, transfers these qualities and virtues to the drinker.

The wine's physiological properties, varying according to the composition of the soil, work on the body and in so doing its soul, which has been thoroughly imbued with them, acts on the psyche of those with the discernment to choose and appreciate it.

The respect shown to the juice of the vine in seeking to improve its quality has played a large part since ancient times in raising humanity from its primitive brutish state. The cultivation of and trade in wine led people to adopt a certain way of life which over the centuries has spread from the shores of the Mediterranean to many other regions. Apart from the recognised medicinal virtues of grape juice, the product of the vine has inspired poets, philosophers and the founders of religion. Homer described wine as 'glowing' because it fuels the blood of man, while for Plato it is a virtual fire that heats the soul and the body. Plato also observes in his *Treatise on Laws* that 'wine is both sacrament and recreation for men of mature years; it was given them by a god as a remedy for the austerity of old age.'

The Civilising Effect of Wine

It is impossible to name all the writers who have sung its praises. We shall therefore confine ourselves to just a few of them.

For the French writer Georges Duhamel (1884–1966), who was also a qualified physician, wine is the prototype of the particular culture which makes up Western thought and moral attitudes. These show themselves in different ways according to the individual character of each wine-growing region, in the same way as wines from the same stock vary according to the nature of the soil that feeds them.

For generations a considered approach to the 'divine nectar' has shaped people's way of life, affecting their personality and so influencing their customs and attitudes. This process has bred an entire literature and dictated its styles of expression. We shall be returning to this in Part Two, in the chapter on the relationship between wine and the psyche.

As for the influence of this 'oenological' culture on social and cultural patterns of life, among the peoples of old Europe we can distinguish individual peculiarities so subtle they are often difficult to pinpoint, just like the nuances of character revealed in vine cultivation and wine consumption. The Rhineland or Mosel character, to give just one example, is closer to the Latin mentality than that of the Bavarians or the Saxons, who prefer beer. As for the Viennese, their nature is surely a reflection of their white wines, produced on the banks of the Danube.

André Maurois believes that these ethical and spiritual attributes, born of a wine-growing civilisation, show themselves in a certain finesse and sensibility. In the cultivation of the vine and the constant search for improvement in the quality of the product, we can see why we should prize so highly such virtues as respect for time, patience in one's work and the cultivation of taste and sound judgement—all of which tend to be neglected today in favour of quantity and profit. When applied to quality control in wine and the maintenance of a stable physiological balance, obeying and following these rules creates a personality in keeping with the beverage itself and achieves harmony between body and spirit. A vintage of good standard, with a soul that rises free of its physical matrix during tasting, cannot be achieved in a hurry. Years of effort and patience are needed to obtain a vine that will produce a wine worthy of the name. Isn't the same true of health? In both cases we must persevere come what may, care about it and feel free to criticise or praise the end result.

Environment and Selection

Before we can respect the wine we drink, we must adopt the right attitude towards it, so that it will respond to our physiological and mental needs in the way we have a right to expect.

After all, we change our clothes to suit the occasion, whether social or professional, and according to the weather and season. Our choice of style, colour and accessories depends on individual taste, and it is in the quality of this choice that we reveal our personalities. It therefore presupposes a selection process. The same holds true for a particular vintage and the way we use it. When we select a wine, our choice involves seeking a balance between the composition of the menu, the quality of the wine and the vintage that will enhance the meal. The resulting harmony intensifies the digestive benefits of the juice of the vine and for that reason alone justifies its place on our table.

It is a strange paradox of the 1990s that, although we in the highly developed countries can now enjoy a much wider variety of foods, our choice of diet is increasingly tied to a regime one can only describe as spartan. To subject ourselves to this type of diet in the name of some ill-conceived notion of healthy living leads to inadequate nutrition and leaves us with a choice of insipid liquids as accompaniments to our wretched feasts: we will call for a carafe of water, if not for drinks made up of chemicals, wrongly praising them as beneficial to health.

These heresies of taste are further compounded by errors concerning quality.

In our age of uniformity and egalitarianism, which has created the 'unisex' look, the physiological needs of the stomach are being satisfied without regard for the gastronomic rules dear to our forebears—which moreover were based on good sense. We should not fall prey to these nutritional aberrations which, in the guise of sophisticated culinary recipes, make the reputation of certain *chefs de cuisine* who actually deserve the title of laboratory technician. We also hear the feeble excuse—only occasionally justifiable—of lack of time as a reason for succumbing to the fashion for fast food, whose ingredients would make the great chefs of the past turn in their graves. To wash down this type of diet, people quench their thirst by reaching for artificially coloured and sweetened liquids which scarcely deserve the name of wine. All in all, why wonder at the resulting indigestion and symptoms of depression that plague these new 'gastronomes.'

In properly prepared foods there is both a physiological and a psychological relationship with the wines that bring out their taste, and this satisfies not only the body but the spirit, the physical and the mental; it creates a feeling of balanced well-being which indicates a state of perfect physical harmony.

Rather than listing all the possible permutations in this association between various dishes and the appropriate beverage, we shall mention just a few by way of example. All the flavour of a true Toulouse cassoulet is brought out by choosing a Cahors wine and that of hot sausage in oil by washing it down with a Beaujolais. Cheeses, too, benefit from a choice of the correct wine. Following the sound advice offered by Maître Pierre Androuet, Roquefort agrees very well with a Sauternes wine and a Saint Nectaire calls for a red Graves.

My purpose here in insisting on the advantages of a correct combination of what we eat and what we drink is to stress the beneficial effects on the entire system, the main agent of which is the product of the vine.

CHAPTER 4

WINE AND THE SENSES

In keeping with the theme of this book, I shall say little about wine from its purely oenological aspect, since that is a matter for specialists. I shall therefore confine myself to matters relating to my capacity as a doctor of medicine. The fermented juice of the vine will be discussed in relation to its function of arousing the different sensory, motory and mental reactions in the consumer during the various phases of its contact with the mucous membranes of the digestive system and the higher nervous centres.

In chapter 3, I pointed out that the product of the vine, initially mere fruit juice with a basis of water and mineral salts, is, after its delicate processing, thanks to the genius of the vine grower, imbued with its own soul. Hidden deep in the bottle, it is apparent to anyone who takes the trouble to look for it. This subtle spirit, plainly visible in those myriads of bubbles effervescing from a bottle of Champagne, comes from its material body. And because of their richness and variety, the components of this vinous body, awakened like Sleeping Beauty by the fermenting process, will set in motion a series of physiological stimuli reverberating right to the centre of the mind. The loop connecting the physical to the mental is thus completed. At every stage in its direct or indirect contact with a part of the body, wine provokes a series of chain reactions in the functions of the part concerned.

Let us look at what happens.

Sight

Gazing at a carafe, even one made of cut crystal, will do nothing for you if it is filled with mere tap water. Looking at the contents will leave you indifferent. It is quite another matter when, even before opening it, you are looking at a good bottle of wine; as Montaigne recommended, 'let your eyes taste it before you sample it.'

The first sensation experienced by the drinker is of a visual order. Your eye is struck by the colours of the liquid, already delectable in themselves, with a chromatic range worthy of the brush of a Van Gogh. In the red wines, the colour scale goes from pure red to ruby, ranging, according to vintage, through violet and garnet. In their turn, the white wines offer a whole palette of yellows, from pale to true amber, with gradations of greenish yellow and gold; and we must not forget the various tints of the rosé wines, clothed in their bright hues.

These colourful vibrations pierce the pupil, impregnate the retina and activate the optic nerve which transmits waves to the vision centres of the brain. Here, transformed into sensitive impressions, they create a feeling of gladness, awaken happy memories and recall lines of poetry, an emotional state which no robot, however perfect, would be capable of feeling and expressing.

Smell

As Pierre Poulon wrote, 'One sees with the nose as one drinks with the eyes.'

In the second stage of the wine ceremony, fill your glass and raise it level with your nostrils to perform the test for a 'bouquet', which is a harmonious blend of odoriferous molecules. The physiological importance of this operation may be gauged from the fact that it has given rise to a form of treatment based on essential oils, aromatherapy. Its medicinal value rests on the arousal of the sense of smell, a sense which must have been one of the first to develop in primitive man, when he was still close to his animal nature. His evolvement gave him closer contact with the outside world. To survive, cave-dwellers had to rely on hunting for their daily food and the search for game required tracking skills.

Having said this, we have to accept that our formerly keen sense of smell has diminished with the advance of civilisation, both mechanical and intellectual. Today, the only use we make of this sense is when we receive everyday odours which are usually more or less agreeable. We no longer have any real appreciation of scents, other than the fragrant outpourings from noble or sophisticated perfumes.

Among these quality aromas, that of good wine, mainly through its esters and aldehydes, is highly favoured by the connoisseur. For the physician, these molecules redolent of the perfumes of fruits, flowers or musk which together make up a wine's bouquet, have a physiological significance. Caught by a bundle of nerve cells lodged in the membrane that coats the inside of the nasal cavities, these elements in their turn set in motion reactions which are communicated directly to the brain. As in the case of vision, the receiving centre, which is next to the pituitary gland, activates it and this affects the entire endocrine system.

Looking at the results obtained from the medicinal uses of essential oils, one might well wonder if, according to the quality and variety of the bouquet, these odoriferous molecules emanating from a quality vintage might not also be capable of playing a certain therapeutic role. In any case, when sniffed by a reasonably knowledgeable lover of wine, who need not be a recognised wine expert, this stimulus transforms the sensory responses into a series of euphoric emotional impressions. The messages received by the nose enrich still further the response already registered by the eyes.

Taste

As a logical consequence of the stages briefly described above in our discussion of the physiological and psychological value of a thoughtful approach to wine, the next stage, during which we drink this noble beverage, will occupy a privileged place because of the functional reactions it will bring about.

Wine is not for swallowing like any old liquid. It must first be warmed by being held for a moment in the mouth and 'chewed'. This slight rise in temperature, particularly with red wines, allows the aromatic elements of the vintage to deploy their whole range of perfumes within the mouth cavity, and so to intensify the work already begun at the 'nasal' stage.

The contact of the wine with the taste buds on the tongue, the mucus on the palate and the sides of the mouth provokes a sensation of physical pleasure which shows itself by an increased secretion of saliva. This reaction is commonly described by the apt expression 'the mouth begins to water'. As for the wine expert, as a connoisseur he appreciates the flavours released for what they are and interprets the whole range at his leisure.

You will find that the flow of saliva, stimulated by the aromatic elements present in the wine, will increase with the age of the bottled vintage you have chosen. This in turn will stimulate a parallel increase in the flow of digestive juices, especially ptyalin, an enzyme which contributes to the partial metabolism of carbohydrates and starchy substances. Seen from this somewhat prosaic angle, the ritual of wine-tasting actually aids the digestive process. Apart from this initial physiological reaction, the effect goes beyond the digestive system itself, for the body's response also affects the mind. Because of their importance and value, we shall come back to the consequences of these different reactions in the chapter on the relationship between wine and the psyche.

CHAPTER 5

WINE DRINKING

In this book we have frequently stressed the importance of an 'intelligent' approach to wine in day-to-day living, if only to counter the disparaging comments of its detractors, who concentrate most of their criticism on its alcohol content. Later on I shall show exactly how much credence should be given to this.

The very fact of drinking wine requires us to follow certain guidelines that will make it a more enjoyable experience as well as being better for us.

From the doctor's point of view—his patients' health—these guidelines apply just as much to the amount one should drink as to the 'quality' of the wine and its selection. I explained my views on this last point in a book dealing with the role of wine in different aspects of our lives and careers and in different states of health.* When we consider its dual role as a dietary and medicinal supplement, we can see that in our dealings with it we should observe certain rules. We need to tailor our choice according to our individual physique and state of health, and to vary this when we are ill. Our own particular temperament (in the Hippocratic sense of the word) is also a factor to consider. This angle, which is quite important, will be the subject of the last part of this book.

* *Notre Vin Quotidien*, Editions Universitaires.

Sensible Drinking

The nutritionists, following in the steps of the health experts, have tried to classify wine as an 'alcoholic' beverage. It is quite true that it contains alcohol, mainly in the form of ethanol, the result of the natural fermentation of the grape, but this should not be confused with the alcohol that is manufactured by distilling. There is a great difference here. Moreover, the respective alcoholic strengths are not at all comparable.

It is therefore quite wrong to think of the fermented juice of the vine as nothing more than diluted alcohol of whatever strength. On the contrary, in natural fermentations the alcohol is enriched by other elements—nitrogenous substances, mineral salts, trace elements and vitamins—which reduce its potentially harmful effects while blending harmoniously with it.

Having made this point, all we have to do is establish guidelines regarding the amount of wine it is wise to drink. This is simple, as they are based on precise physiological data.

Whatever its origin, alcohol that accumulates in the body has harmful effects; if one exceeds the acceptable dose, it then impregnates the body tissues, causing damage to their cells. To be tolerated, ingested alcohol must be metabolised—that is, transformed by oxidation. This latter process cannot go beyond what the system can cope with. The chemical transformation of ethanol takes place in the liver through the action of an enzyme, dehydrogenase, which transforms the alcohol in the wine by decomposing it, but under certain conditions and within certain limits. This will be discussed in more detail later. Determining these parameters can be compared with the process that determines the choice and dosage of pharmaceutical drugs and monitors their effects. A particular dose of active ingredients is beneficial to the invalid. Beyond that it becomes toxic; below that, ineffective.

The same is true for the fermented juice of the vine and its dosage. Reading these lines, any wine expert will protest that our association with the 'divine nectar' cannot possibly be compared to the mere taking of some medicine or other. However, my reply to that is that since the theme of this book is derived from the teachings of Hippocrates, we are reasoning here as followers of the Master of Cos—hence the need to establish a specific dosage.

The acceptable amount for a healthy adult taking moderate physical exercise is equivalent to the ratio of one gramme of wine-alcohol per kilo of weight per day. In theory, according to Charles Fiessinger, an individual weighing, say, 70 kilos (11 stone) and eating a balanced diet, can absorb daily a maximum of one litre of wine at 10 per cent strength, when this quantity is divided equally between the two main meals. For manual workers, who need a higher calorie intake, especially if they are exposed to bad weather, this dose may be increased. But normally, in view of the sedentary life most of us lead nowadays, wisdom dictates that we should limit ourselves to three quarters of a litre of wine at 11 per cent strength, taking half this amount with each of the two main meals of the day. For women, the optimum amount over the twenty-four hours should not exceed half a litre.

These established data can offer a rough guide which should be kept in mind.

Individual Tolerance Thresholds

These ratios vary according to the alcohol level found in the particular vintage selected. It is quite obvious that, without harmful consequences to health, one cannot consume during the course of a day the amount of wine indicated above if the alcohol level exceeds 12 per cent. Furthermore, even when keeping within the permitted limits, we cannot ignore a second factor: our individual tolerance thresholds to wine, which are different for each of us.

In his or her approach to the fermented juice of the grape, the consumer should bear in mind three factors. The first, of a physiological nature, concerns the sensory stimuli activated during any absorption of liquids, in this case wine. The organic responses vary considerably and I have dealt with this subject in chapter 4. The second factor is chemical and concerns the relationship between the components of the wine and the quality of the food eaten. As for the last factor, and it is no less important, this is the 'spiritual' feeling awakened by the enjoyment of the wine. We shall return to this aspect of the discussion later.

Looking at it another way, assuming that wine can be prescribed medicinally for anyone who, without being seriously ill, must nevertheless follow a special diet, disregarding the 'great wines' your preference should be for vintages coming from old vines, which are richer in reserves. In the case of the white wines of Alsace, Jura, Savoy or the Loire Valley, these must have an alcohol level equal to or higher than 8.5 per cent. As for red wines, their alcohol content must not exceed 15 per cent. Moreover their acidity, in the form of tartaric acid, must be at least 4.5g per litre. A good number of table wines answer to these conditions.

Having said that, how should we go about this commonplace daily routine which, if we respect it, will ensure that our association with the 'divine nectar' will do us no harm?

Drinking Know-how

After briefly lingering in the mouth cavity and triggering off physiological reactions, the wine goes down into the stomach. If the stomach cavity is empty, the ingested liquid passes through the pylorus (the opening into the duodenum) too quickly. In less than half an hour, the components of the wine make their way into the blood-stream. As for the ethanol, it passes to the liver to be oxidised there.

When the stomach is empty this mechanical process is speeded up and the liver then has to perform its function in a hurry. The available dehydrogenase will not be sufficient to cope and the alcohol, its molecules still not broken down, will be absorbed by the other body tissues, chiefly those of the central nervous system. In such a scenario, the strength of the alcohol remains the same and becomes harmful to the system. Its consequences are only too well known—some immediate, such as a state of inebriation, others more long term but boding ill for future health.

On the other hand, if before any wine is swallowed the stomach is ballasted with food, even a small amount, the pylorus relaxes more slowly, opening gradually to allow the passage of food particles. The flow of liquid towards the duodenum is thus slowed down. The liver has time to carry out the oxidisation of the ethanol and so diminishes the effects of the ethyl complex. Plain common sense therefore dictates that we should not drink any wine on an empty stomach. From the physiological point of view, the best time to enjoy the 'divine nectar' is during meals. This might seem a blindingly obvious remark, but I don't think it a waste of time to mention it for the sake of those who, at every opportunity and at any time of the day, sacrifice to Bacchus.

On certain business or social occasions we may find

ourselves obliged (very agreeably, one might say) to start with a drink containing some degree of alcohol as an apéritif—that is, with the aim of stimulating the appetite. In these circumstances we should plump for an extra-dry Champagne, the most suitable vintage for such situations. Following the rule laid down above, care should be taken to accompany it by nibbling a few cocktail snacks and, out of respect for the wine itself, to savour it in little sips. The bouquet will be better appreciated and, physiologically speaking, the digestive process will work more efficiently.

Eating Know-how

'Eating know-how' goes hand in hand with 'drinking know-how'. This aspect of the art of living has nothing to do with the results of certain present-day culinary research, which often has more in common with chemistry than with the harmonious blending of nutritious ingredients. The happy marriage of food and drink contributes in large measure to improving the body's tolerance with regard to the effects of wine alcohol. This joint action has its place within the framework of an intelligent diet based on a balanced food intake and a sensible choice of vintage to complete this ensemble. It is not a question here of gastronomy, but rather of guidelines for healthy eating.

A meal accompanied by wine must accordingly include plenty of foods containing glucids and lipids. Among the first we can count vegetables and fruits; among the second, products rich in animal or vegetable fats. I would point out in passing that the consumption of red meats lowers the alcohol level in the blood by 10 to 20 per cent. This fact might be of interest to the car driver planning to get behind the wheel after dining too well.

There are other constituents of a meal rich in natural

vitamins which contribute in their turn to the body's greater tolerance of wine. These substances are found in the elements that make up the vitamin B complex. They function through their protective action by means of thiamine, which is also used in the medical treatment of illnesses caused by ethyl impregnation. Any deficiency of this group of vitamins increases the body's sensitivity to the effects of wine alcohol. It can therefore be made good by including in the daily diet (particularly at breakfast) foods rich in cereals of all kinds, such as barley, wheat germ and especially by regularly eating wholemeal or brown bread.

These are some of the rules you should follow to ensure that the wine accompanying your meal remains, as Louis Pasteur has so rightly claimed, 'the healthiest and the most health-giving of drinks.'

Let the Spirit Breathe . . .

Finally, we must be sure to fulfil one last condition in order that the 'divine nectar', fully savoured, may rejoice our hearts without damaging our health at all. This condition concerns our emotional side.

Because of its importance, I shall be returning to this subject at greater length at the end of Part Two of this book. For the moment, let us remain at the more humdrum level of daily living.

The irregular rhythm of modern life in the big urban and suburban centres forces most people living in them to eat out at least once a day. This basic need is satisfied most often in a hurry, amid jostling crowds, noise and tobacco smoke. Not only that, the fare on offer in the canteen or the cheaper cafés includes poor quality wine of doubtful origin, unless people resort to drowning their food in those reputedly 'healthy' drinks (because they are 'alcohol-free') based on chemical products, which are certainly more toxic than a few grammes of wine alcohol. In some quarters, in the grip of a new gastronomic craze, people fall for the cult of fast food, which means swallowing at record speed foods pre-cooked in the bowels of vast industrial kitchens. This style of eating accords ill with the agreeable enjoyment of wine that benefits the whole system.

In both cases, these factors, accumulating over time, eventually affect the balance of the autonomic nervous system, which has already been upset by the environmental assaults of noise and lights. The effect of these physical factors has repercussions at an emotional level, so leading to a condition of stress which the victim may or may not be aware of. In addition, the digestive function is impaired, and this plays a part in lowering the body's tolerance threshold to wine. In the lifestyle described above, it is therefore better to do without wine and wait until it can be enjoyed in a more favourable atmosphere. With luck the home environment will offer this opportunity, but only if you do not indulge in the detestable habit of eating your evening meal facing a television screen.

The author of these snippets of advice, which he believes are based on good sense, is aware that he is preaching in the wilderness. Nevertheless, he will stay the course, refusing to betray his physician's calling and his dual role of dispenser of wisdom and wine enthusiast.

PART TWO
WINE AND THE FUNCTIONS

'If I were asked what, of earth's bounty, takes pride of place,
I would say, it is wine.'

Cato the Elder

A ban on so-called alcoholic drinks is routine practice whenever people are put on a diet for the sake of their health, if not by their doctor, at least by a qualified dietician.

This restriction is perfectly understandable, but the snag is that the ban usually includes wine drinking.

Throughout this book I have been at pains to prove that, at risk of being accused of ignorance or dishonesty, one cannot include the fermented juice of the vine in this category. As we have already noted, the ethanol in wine, the result of a natural chemical transformation within the sugary elements of the grape, should not be confused with alcohol, which is the artificial substitute produced by distillation.

To debar a sick person from enjoying an honest vintage in reasonable doses and above all chosen to suit his specific condition (apart from exceptions of which his doctor is the sole judge) is sometimes the result of ignorance of the medicinal benefits that wine can provide. In other cases it may stem from a sort of nutritional snobbery of an emotional nature. In neither case is there any scientific basis for the ban, as has several times been proved by leading clinicians whose authority and good faith are beyond question. The numerous clinical trials they have conducted were referred to in Part One, chapter 2.

Besides, it is not that long ago that the Pharmacopoeia included in its official prescriptions a whole range of medicinal wines for therapeutic use adapted to the various needs of the sick. To name a few, there was *Vin de Trousseau* containing digitalis for cardiac cases, the wine produced by La Charité, enriched with squill for the treatment of kidney failure, wines rich in iron for anaemia, onion wines to help prostate problems.

By its very nature and because of the natural ingredients that make it up, wine can be regarded as a food, a physical and mental tonic, an aid to digestion, a mineral supplement, an antibiotic, an anti-allergic agent. It provides vitamins, regulates the system, and we must not forget its preventative and stabilising effect on the whole of the cardiovascular system.

There is therefore quite a close link between the main physiological functions of the body and the potential effect on them of wine drinking if they fail to work properly. However, the juice of the vine should not be regarded as a substitute for medicines. Nevertheless, thanks to the elements it supplies to the body, it is capable of playing the role of medical 'auxiliary', in conjunction with the other remedies prescribed by the doctor.

The development of this argument will form the subject of Part Two of this book.

CHAPTER 1
WINE AND DIGESTION

At the risk of being accused of stating the blindingly obvious, it must be said that, in our part of the world, it is normal practice for the wine bottle to appear on the table twice a day when people sit down to satisfy the natural demands of their stomachs.

In countries where oenology (the study of wine) has an honoured place, people would not dream of eating a meal, however modest, without the accompaniment of one or more glasses of the potion that is sacred to Bacchus. Apart from the pleasure they get from this custom, in practice it has a beneficial effect on the digestive mechanism. We have already stressed the point that a meal washed down with tap water, even if it is served in a crystal carafe, is an unfortunate error in taste and a grave dietary error, as it is one of the causes of dyspepsia. Relying on this tasteless beverage affects the elasticity of the stomach cavity and changes the catalytic value (the ability to break down foods) of the digestive juices, apart from its negative influence at a psychological level which, in the habitual water drinker, may encourage a tendency to pessimism and introspection.

In Part One, chapter 4 of this book, we alluded to the influence of the sensory stimuli on the flow of digestive secretions. But this action does not just stop at the mouth cavity. It extends throughout the alimentary canal and gives rise to other reactive phenomena, sometimes even taking on a medicinal role.

Wine as Food

Certain people who are badly informed, if not actually prejudiced, have cast doubt on the nutritional value of wine. To them the product of the grape is nothing more than a kind of liquid, and seeing only its physical aspect, they regard it as a watery solution with a pleasant taste, but which may, eventually, prove toxic to those who drink it.

It is worth reminding these kindly detractors of what Olivier de Serres noted in his book published in 1660, *Le Théâtre de l'Agriculture*: 'After bread comes wine, the second food given by the Creator to maintain life and the first celebrated for its excellence.'

Echoing this author, the learned Italian Baglioni commented that the fermented juice of the vine belongs, together with oil and bread, to that trilogy of foods deified by Greek mythology.

Endorsing the opinion of these two agronomists, recent analyses carried out by researchers and dieticians have proved that a good quality wine is likely to supply about a quarter of the body's calorie requirements (about 700 to 800). Apart from the glucidic content due to the presence of ethanol, the level of which varies according to degree between 45 and 160 grammes per litre, this beverage contains, according to the latest analyses, around 600 identifiable components which, in terms of food value, mean that it is certainly a source of the nutrients that help to sustain life.

Wine, a living liquid of unchanging composition, can therefore be assessed as an additional, digestible source of food. Other than water and alcohol, it contains sugar, glycerine, amino and organic acids, mineral salts, proteins and gelatinous matter. As for glycerol, a polyalcohol present in wine, and natural phosphates, these combine in the body with the glycerine normally already present in the intestine to form glycerophosphates, a storing medium for the whole system. For this reason alone the juice of the vine forms an alternative, complementary food, reducing the body's need for carbohydrates—which shows the place that a correctly chosen wine can occupy in the diet of the diabetic. We shall be returning to this in the chapter on the role of wine in the functioning of the metabolism.

Wine as Appetiser

The fermented juice of the vine is rightly thought of as an appetiser, and it should be your preferred choice for this purpose. Sipped before sitting down at the table, it whets the appetite instead of spoiling it, as is the case when one falls for the snobbery of high-alcohol concoctions, abuse of which can lead to alcoholic saturation.

However, for wine to fulfil the function of appetiser without having any long-term effects on the consumer's health, it is important to make your choice from the most appropriate vintages. Some of those classified as sweet apéritif wines are too high in alcohol to be used on a regular basis. You would do better to choose one of the light white, rather dry wines such as extra-dry Champagne which is heartily recommended for several reasons. There is no point in dwelling on the oenological aspect, which needs no comment. But from the dietary point of view, this wine has a beneficial effect on the alimentary canal through its natural aeration. This acts on the stomach muscles which thus retain their suppleness and elasticity. The expulsion of gases through the mouth (preferably as discreetly as possible if you are in polite company) bears witness to this. The only drawback to this choice of wine is the rather heavy burden it places on the purse, especially if you intend to make a habit of it. To get round this monetary obstacle while achieving, albeit to a lesser degree, the same goal, you might try, depending on personal taste, the Gaillac sparkling wines or the light, sparkling wines of Die.

But whatever the circumstances and whatever vintage you select, you must be careful to give your body time to metabolise the ethanol. The reasons for this were given in the previous chapter. So while sipping the vintage of your choice, provide a few cocktail snacks to eat at the same time.

Wine and the Stomach

A good quality wine, taken in reasonable amounts during the meal, improves the working of the stomach through its digestive properties. There is a story that Saint Paul, apostle of the gentiles, once gave this very good advice to one of his disciples who suffered from indigestion: 'Drink no longer water, but use a little wine for thy stomach's sake and thine often infirmities' (1 Tim. 5:23).

We have several times stressed that the fermented juice of the vine cannot be regarded as a tame beverage for quenching the thirst. According to the variety of vine, its 'bouquet' delights both the drinker's sense of smell and his sense of taste. Without claiming to be a gourmet, it must be agreed that eating a healthy and enjoyable diet is not simply a matter of establishing the right balance in the intake of essential foods. That approach belongs to the category of what one might describe as 'joyless dietetics'. It is equally important to relish what we eat and to do this we need to add something to our meal that will enhance the flavour of the food on our plate. Only a good wine, chosen not merely to complement the food but also to suit the needs of the individual, will provide the right stimulation. This does away with the need for other artificial digestive agents which, if they become a habit, may eventually irritate the stomach lining.

While acting as a seasoning, wine is also good for the digestive process. On contact with the stomach, it stimulates the production of digestive juices. Experiments have shown that swallowing 60 to 100 grammes of wine results in a secretion of 100 to 120 grammes of liquid containing around a gramme of free hydrochloric acid. The assimilation of proteins is made easier by this state of ionic acidity and by the gentle osmotic pressure exercised on the stomach wall. Finally, in the opinion of Doctor Marchal, the ingestion of sweet white wines enriches the gastric juice by an influx of white corpuscles, acting then as an oxidising ferment to encourage the metabolism of albuminoid substances such as meat and especially fish. This latter property would explain, physiologically speaking, why we naturally select white wines to accompany a menu consisting of fish, whether fresh-water or sea fish.

Apart from these stimulating and digestive functions, wine also supplies certain B complex vitamins, such as riboflavin and pantothenic acid, which help in the metabolism of proteins and glucides.

WINE AND INDIGESTION

The above observations assume that the stomach is working normally. But there are many people with a delicate nervous system who may have some difficulty in tolerating wine. In such cases, the choice of vintage will depend on what is wrong with them. As a complement to any medicine that has been prescribed, the wine selected should act as a medicinal auxiliary, and your choice should be made with this in mind.

I have already commented that the wines from the Champagne region, whether dry or extra-dry, have a beneficial effect, both chemical and mechanical, on the digestive system. They are therefore recommended for people suffering from flatulence (aerophagia) and a bloated stomach. The potassium tartrate they contain helps to contract and tone the muscular fibres of the stomach wall. On the other hand, the presence of natural carbonic acid revives the organ's elasticity. The formation of gases resulting from the slow fermentation process of these vintages differs from the artificially created gases resulting from the crude techniques used in the manufacture of certain sparkling wines. It is not surprising that this type of drink causes a build-up of gases in the stomach and intestines, which is not the case with the wines of Champagne. When taken for this purpose by those suffering from aerophagia, who are often of a nervous disposition, they should not exceed the recommended dose of one or two glasses ten minutes before the meal.

STOMACH PAINS

In contrast to the foregoing, there are some people who suffer from heartburn, often caused by a temperament that is prone to anxiety and easily upset. In consequence, the stomach contracts and secretes an excessive amount of hydrochloric acid.

To alleviate these problems, sufferers from stomach pains should restrict their choice, according to personal taste if not the composition of the menu, to red or white wines which are low in acidity and rich in calcium, such as the wines of Anjou or the Saumurois. They may also drink the wines of Sauternes or Barsac. Through the calcium salts they contain, these still, sweet and soft wines have a stabilising and sedative effect on the sympathetic nervous system. No more than one or two glasses should be drunk with meals, and the menu should be chosen to take account of digestive difficulties; your doctor or dietician will advise you on this aspect of the problem.

POOR MUSCLE TONE

There is one final condition that may also require treatment with the appropriate choice of wine. Although there is no wind or bloating, the digestive process may be slowed down as a result of a certain sluggishness due to poor muscle tone in the stomach area, which leads to some deficiency in gastric secretions.

To remedy this situation, you should make your choice, according to individual taste, either from the wines of Monbazillac, or from those of the Médoc. The former will act through their content of calcium salts and magnesium which will tone up the sympathetic nervous system controlling the function of the gastro-intestinal apparatus. As for the wines of the Médoc, rich in iron, phosphates and tannin, when drunk with meals their role as a tonic will be quite significant. Taken in moderation (two glasses twice a day during meals), they will give the stomach wall greater elasticity, speeding up the digestion of food.

CONSTIPATION

The action of the fermented juice of the vine is not limited to the stage of gastric digestion. Once through the pylorus (the opening between the stomach and the duodenum), it starts to affect the intestines by regularising, according to the wine chosen, the secretory and motor mechanisms of this section of the alimentary canal.

As an experiment, Loeper and his colleagues asked a volunteer patient to swallow the equivalent of 20 cubic centimetres of a sweet wine from the Vouvray region. Afterwards, by passing a tube into the duodenum, they were able to collect 120 grammes of pure bile. This result confirms the action of sweet white wines on the functioning of the gall bladder in increasing the volume of bile secretion. For people suffering from a certain intestinal sluggishness, the sweet white wines of the Anjou region, rich in glycerol and sorbitol, will relieve constipation in the same way as Epsom salts, without the drawbacks of the latter due to their violent effects and the nasty taste they leave in the mouth. The only restriction on this form of wine therapy is that it should be avoided by diabetics, the obese and those suffering from high blood pressure.

On average, a quarter of a bottle per meal is an effective and reasonable dose.

DIARRHOEA

We shall be returning later to the rich tannin content of the Médoc wines and their effect on the circulation. Remaining for the present with the digestion and the matter of choosing wines suitable for diarrhoea sufferers, these Médoc wines will work on the problem through their richness in tannin. This product tones up the smooth intestinal muscles and helps to restore the rhythm of contractions. To take an example, as a historical footnote, it is worth recalling the case of the Duc de Richelieu, at that time Governor of Guyenne. This illustrious personage complained to his doctor of a certain 'languor of the intestines', a phenomenon which could be compared in our day to a form of inflammation of the colon. The wise doctor he consulted, who must have been a wine expert, advised him to drink the wines of the Médoc with his meals. His patient's return to health, thanks to this clever bit of wine medication, led to these vintages being honoured with the title 'Tisane de Richelieu'.

Putting the astringent properties of tannin to good use, the Médoc vintages will have a place on the tables of those whose digestion is too rapid, particularly when this phenomenon is followed by a chill affecting the abdominal region: in short, these vintages should be part of the menu of those suffering from diarrhoea, who should drink the equivalent of half a bottle a day.

WINE LIST

Vintages	Clinical Indications
Champagne (extra-dry) Gaillac perlé Clairette de Die	Appetite (loss of)
Champagne (extra-dry)	Indigestion
Barsac Sauternes	Stomach pains
Médoc Monbazillac	Sluggish stomach
Anjou (sweet white) Bandol Bergerac Vouvray (sweet white)	Constipation
Médoc Madizan	Diarrhoea and Gastro-enteritis

CHAPTER 2
WINE AND THE CIRCULATION

Before discussing the beneficial effect of particular wines on the state of the arteries and consequently on that of the heart muscles, I should like to draw attention to a recent inquiry carried out by some British researchers (Doctors Streger, Cochrane and Moore), whose impartiality cannot be doubted. The researchers reached the conclusion that people living in wine-growing countries, and therefore habitual wine drinkers, were less prone to cardiovascular disease than those from beer-drinking regions or those who preferred soft drinks. A recent survey conducted by the *New Journal of Medicine* on a total of 100,000 women threw light on the preventative effect of wine alcohol in relation to myocardial infarction (heart attacks). Similarly, researchers at the Harvard Medical School also produced statistics showing that the risk of heart attack is greater among non-wine drinkers. According to these researchers, the ethanol in the wine has an effect on cholesterol and on the process of platelet aggregation which plays an important part in the formation of clots.

This work merely confirms that of Professor Masquelier, whose work will be discussed at greater length later in this chapter.

Long before these experts, Dr Noel Fiessinger (1881–1946), good clinician that he was, had observed in his turn that cases of arterial atheroma (fatty degeneration of the arteries) were found less frequently among habitual wine drinkers. In this brief survey of the importance granted by doctors to the fermented juice of the vine as auxiliary medication in cardiac or arterial complaints, reference has been made to the effect of wine on the heart and the arteries, and this is given added weight by the phytotherapists, who long ago used the medicinal virtues of the black grape, rich in pigments and tannin, to deal with problems in the veins, from varicose veins to haemorrhoids.

Causes and Consequences

The experimental work of Professor Masquelier and his colleagues has confirmed the protective power of wine for people suffering from arteriosclerosis and its consequences. This medicinal effect is due not, as was first thought, to the presence in wine of ethyl alcohol, but to the amount of procyanidines in grape juice, elements which are found in the pips of the woody part of the grape cluster. Furthermore, these same products also play a part in treating other diseases that affect the circulatory system.

The process of progressive degeneration of the walls of the arteries which, sooner or later, leads to arteriosclerosis, can have several causes. It may be linked to the person's age, to bad eating habits, to a sedentary lifestyle—things which, like arthritis symptoms, people usually allow to develop before they try to do anything about them.

Without dwelling any longer on the causes, let us confine ourselves to the biological facts revealed by the researchers mentioned above, which will help us to understand the beneficial effect of wine.

Any injury affecting the arterial wall encourages a local build-up of cholesterol which is then found in the blood at a somewhat higher level. Hence, weakness in the vascular wall leads to an excessive local increase in histamine, a product which contributes to the widening of the capillaries and increases the production of organic secretions. This factor is at the basis of allergic symptoms, such as hives. (In this connection, it should be pointed out that Doctor Weisseimbach recommended patients who were allergic to strawberries to soak the fruit beforehand in a bowl of red wine). The histamine then makes the arterial wall more permeable to other lipidic elements. Here and there it stimulates a proliferation of muscular cells and this reactive mechanism promotes the formation of plaques composed of calcareous deposits and fibrous growth, which we call atheroma. This condition contributes to a further reduction in the diameter of the artery, causing the formation of blood clots, which lead to heart attacks.

It is not the role of this book to dictate the preventative measures we should take, but even so, we should be careful to follow an appropriate dietary regime and a way of life adapted to our condition. Remember that, from the prophylactic point of view, we are concerned with strengthening the arterial wall and avoiding an excessive production of histamine. Our aim is therefore to rejuvenate the tissues of the circulatory system as far as we can.

Pigments and Mineral Salts

After this simplified sketch of the clinical features of arteriosclerosis it remains to decide what place the fermented juice of the vine might occupy in it.

J. Masquelier and his colleagues stressed that wine, and especially red wine, contain, depending on the method of fermentation, a high level of procynanides, whose protective properties for the walls of the veins we mentioned above. To these we can add the beneficial effect of other components of wine, in particular two vitamins. Vitamin C (ascorbic acid) helps to lower the cholesterol level and vitamin P (rutin) regulates the permeability of the blood capillaries, so preventing the transudation of blood plasma. Working with these vitamin sources, wine's mineral salts also play their part. Magnesium exercises anti-coagulant effects and prevents the formation of vascular thrombosis; potassium, in the form of bitartrate, by far the most important in terms of quantity, promotes, according to Laubry, the dilatation of the blood vessels and restores tone and contractility to the heart muscles. Finally, silicium contributes to the homogeneity of the blood vessel walls. Recently, chemical analyses have detected the presence of chromium in wine, at the rate of 450 microgrammes per litre. This metal acts on the metabolism of lipids and glucids, so making it a prophylactic factor in the treatment of arteriosclerosis.

To conclude this short investigation it would be wrong to claim that the juice of the vine, so decried by some health experts, is bad for those suffering degeneration of the arteries. But in order for this beverage to be beneficial, let me reiterate that it should be chosen judiciously and drunk without exceeding the therapeutic limits.

The Choice of Wine

Faced with the symptoms that impair the functioning of the circulatory system, what wines will figure among those recommended by the medical wine waiter?

As an everyday table wine, the diagnosed arteriosclerosis sufferer, or potential sufferer (it is for his doctor to monitor his condition), will prefer the red wines of the Bordeaux region and more particularly those of the Médoc. Indeed, the latter supply these patients with the vitamins they need, and especially with oenotannins which, through the properties described earlier, help strengthen the walls of the blood vessels.

The same wine also plays some part in purging the blood of cholesterol and slowing down the production of histamine.

This choice of wines can be extended further in that the arteriosclerosis sufferer may, from time to time, allow himself an extra supply of magnesium and silicium salts by turning to the wines of the St-Emilion region. The soil there is rich in these mineral salts.

Whatever the wine chosen, the dose of two wine glasses per meal should not be exceeded.

Apart from this basic wine diet, you should bear in mind the complications associated with this condition: arterial hypertension, the risk of narrowing of the coronary arteries and the possibility of a heart attack. In any of these circumstances and irrespective of the treatment given by your doctor or consultant, your diet should be complemented by natural elements designed to strengthen the action of the heart and improve kidney function. You should therefore include the wines of the Champagne region, the extra-dry Champagnes of the Montagne de Reims, Côtes des Blancs or those of the Marne valley.

Without dwelling on the ability of these wines to lift the spirits due to their richness in phosphatic salts—a far from negligible factor for the drinker's state of mind—these wines, through other ingredients, help to maintain the heart muscles and make the arteries more supple. They are rich in magnesium and potassium (from 30 to 100 mg per litre). This latter element, in the form of bitartrate, acts on the heart mechanism and helps to slow down the process of sclerosis of the circulatory system. Furthermore, the sulphuric anions in Champagne wines activate the mechanisms of cellular oxidisation and give them purifying and cleansing properties. Finally, as dry white wines they possess powerful diuretic agents, helping to rid the body of its wastes. All these advantages mean that the wines of this region play an active part in the overall treatment of cardiovascular ailments.

Apart from times of crisis when their medicinal properties can prove highly beneficial, these wines should be used with discretion as a prophylactic measure and only for limited periods. Thus on average you should allow yourself a quarter of a bottle per meal one week in every month; this represents the therapeutically active dose.

WINE LIST

Vintages	Clinical Indications
Médoc St-Emilion	Arteriosclerosis
Champagne (extra-dry) Alsace wines	Arterial hypertension Myocardial infarction (heart attack)

CHAPTER 3

WINE AND ELIMINATION

If one of the effects of taking fresh grapes during the grape cure is to clear the urine of impurities and increase the volume produced, it follows that drinking dry white wines will also increase the quality and volume of this process of elimination, and indeed they have been used for this purpose since remote times.

Virtues of White Wine

Hippocrates, who was one of the first physicians to recognise a definite medicinal value in the fermented juice of the vine, even then prescribed dry white wine to patients suffering from dropsy. Nearer our own time, we should once more recall the wine cures followed by Montaigne, to combat his tendency to accumulate urinary sand in the kidneys. And quite recently, a doctor who was also a wine expert, practising in a town situated on the shores of Lake Geneva, prescribed a cure based on the wines of Crépy to patients who came to consult him about their urinary problems. He was thus competing with the mineral waters of Evian, but the results obtained by this doctor were, it seems, excellent. Here I would comment that the similarity in medicinal properties existing between wine cultivated in this region and the local waters feeding the thermal springs could be explained by the geological nature of the original soil. The same mineral salts with alkalinising properties are present in the soil and pass just as easily into the fruit of the vine as into the ground water feeding the springs.

However, variations exist in the eliminatory action exercised by white wine on the kidneys, differences which relate to the actual composition of the particular wine. The diuretic properties of a Barsac or Sauternes wine are less pronounced than those of the wines of Alsace or Savoy. Like the wines chosen for digestive disorders, those suitable as auxiliaries in the medical treatment of ailments of the urinary system must also be chosen carefully.

How White Wine Works

Like any functioning mechanism, the body has a natural tendency to foul up. The metabolic processes that ensure the maintenance of life ultimately end in the formation of wastes which have to be got rid of in order to avoid a blockage in the machine. Those elements that have become unwanted are the result of physical and chemical processes affecting the protein supply. If they are insufficiently converted, due to a certain sluggishness in the metabolic processes, they then become a source of poisoning, localised in the tissues of the locomotory and eliminatory systems. These residues then take the form of urate or oxalate crystals which lodge either in the joints or in the urinary canals and passages. The result for the individual concerned is painful joints, of which an attack of gout is one example, or urinary sand which can cause attacks of renal colic.

It is understandable, then, that among people susceptible to this ailment or already its victims, it is advisable to cleanse the internal systems from time to time and restore a certain measure of alkalinity to the body. This is achieved by taking a course of diuretic beverages, either in the form of specific mineral waters, or by using an infusion of medicinal plants with eliminatory properties. Among the latter we can include the fruit of the vine, with the proviso that this action is even more apparent if its juice has undergone fermentation and is then drunk in this form. Dry white wine thus plays its part in the biological economy because of its natural acidity and mineral content.

Where Wine is Not Advised . . .

Dry white wines, in spite of their diuretic properties and in fact because of them, are not always suitable for people suffering from urinary complaints, as the eliminatory properties of these wines might lead one to suppose.

Their use is contra-indicated, to give one example, in the case of an illness affecting the organs that secrete or excrete urine, accompanied by sudden rises in temperature, as in acute nephritis (inflammation of the kidneys), urethritis (inflammation of the urethra), or cystitis. One should totally abstain from this type of wine while the inflammation persists. The same line of conduct should also be followed in cases of urinary retention, linked to congestion of the prostate, which leads to an excess of urine in the bladder. It is quite clear that, in each of these cases, medical advice should be sought.

On the other hand, if the wine diet is in question in cases of sudden rises in temperature and pains affecting the joints (I shall be returning at greater length to this subject in a later chapter), it would be best to avoid dry white wines, in favour of red wines not exceeding 9 to 10 per cent.

Apart from these cases, meals can be accompanied by light wines, preferably red, low in alcohol and diluted with a diuretic mineral water.

The real medicinal use for the vintages mentioned at the beginning of this chapter is in the various forms of poisoning of arthritic origin: formation of mineral crystals with its consequences, kidney stones, nephritis (apart from painful attacks) and problems with joints aggravated by changes in humidity.

In all these clinical conditions, the choice of appropriate wine is relatively wide. It depends, as usual, on the patient's individual symptoms.

The Choice of Wine

As a diuretic pure and simple, the best choice is a Muscadet, a wine of low acidity and rich in potassium.

If, on the other hand, there is a more marked tendency for body fluids to be blocked, by urate or oxalate crystals lodged in the joints or urinary tract, it would be better to consider the dry white wines of the region of Sancerre or Pouilly-sur-Loire. They alkalinise the system through the alkaline carbonates they contain and encourage the excretion of urine through their sulphate and potassium tartrate content.

If the presence of kidney stones has been diagnosed clinically and by X-ray, you should try (except during painful attacks) the dry white wines of the Savoy region, Crépy or Ripaille, which are the most diuretic of all the wines of France. To follow the wine cure, you should take one of these two wines at the rate of half a bottle a day, shared between the two main meals. This cure period should not, on average, exceed a fortnight, but may be resumed one or two months later, still following the same dosage and regime.

As a complement to these different choices of wine and to make them even more effective, from time to time it is worth sampling another dry white wine, extra-dry Champagne, which has already been mentioned several times for its medicinal properties. An important reason for this choice, though it is expensive but effective nevertheless, is its richness in potassium tartrate which has great diuretic properties. Apart from this effect, the cleansing action of this type of wine is reinforced by its sulphurous anion content. This element has an eliminatory action on intracellular organic toxins. The centrifugal action of the sulphur thus successfully complements that of the mineral salts cited above and makes the process of organic detoxification more complete. From time to time, over the course of a week, you could allow yourself a daily dose of one or two glasses of this sparkling wine, choosing one that is extra dry, sipping it ten minutes or so before sitting down at table. And there is nothing to stop you remaining faithful to this divine potion throughout the meal.

WINE LIST

Vintages	Clinical Indications
Chablis Muscadet Pouilly Sancerre	Simple urinary problems
Crépy Ripaille	Kidney stones
Champagne extra-dry	Detoxification

CHAPTER 4
WINE AND THE JOINTS

In this account of the influence of the fermented product of the vine on the different parts of the body and their functioning, it is only logical to include the medicinal effects of this beverage on the joints when the latter are anatomically damaged, as is the case in rheumatic conditions. From the form they take, some of these conditions seem to have coincided with the appearance of *Homo erectus*. This means that they are therefore very old and persistent since, even today, they affect about three million people in France alone.

There is no point here in agonising over the possible causes—I leave that to the experts. All I will say is that the whole subject of chronic arthritis, its symptoms and progression, comes under a heading known as 'arthropathy', or genetic predisposition to arthritis.

Before we get to the heart of the matter, we should first make a point concerning diet. There is absolutely no question of condemning the sufferer from chronic rheumatism to drink nothing but tap water at table. Just like any healthy person, he is allowed to drink the juice of the vine with the main proviso that he does so sensibly, but also that he knows which vintage to choose according to his type of rheumatism. A brief look at the clinical aspects will explain the reasons for recommending particular wines.

Rheumatic Symptoms

The different symptoms that appear in the area around

the joints generally have two causes. The first stems from inflammation, complicated by sudden, quite severe rises in temperature. It therefore presents either in the classic form of rheumatic fever or, less severely and following a different course, by an identical inflammation of the joints, which characterises the attacks of arthritis as they gradually develop into a chronic condition.

The second type of rheumatism, by far the most common, stems from the body's actual constitution. In other words, there is a genetic tendency for it to develop. The person affected by it suffers from varying degrees of pain which is aggravated by movement and in particular by changes in air humidity or by being in a humid environment. This type of rheumatism also causes functional problems which may cripple the sufferer.

Finally, there is a form that is progressive, in which the affected joints may become stiff and misshapen: osteoarthritis. This disease affects the connective tissue covering the bone surface and may be considered a kind of localised ageing.

For the moment I shall leave aside that form of hereditary arthritis, gout, the oenological treatment of which will be given in the chapter on the role of wine in metabolic disorders.

Having established these clinical differences, it should be borne in mind that hereditary arthritis does not immediately show itself in its most severe form. In many cases it affects quite a wide range of people who experience such mild and fleeting pains in their joints that they can be classed with those suffering from mild rheumatism. The latter seem to remain free of any serious joint problems and do not suffer any significant functional problems. Only violent movements or changes in temperature cause sudden pain.

Each of these different types of rheumatism requires

the wine drinker to choose from among the most suitable wines to meet his particular case. This choice should be based on the dominant clinical factors and on the constituents of the appropriate vintage. The object of this exercise is to avoid exacerbating the rheumatic condition and to delay its progression as far as possible by supplying any mineral or vitamin deficiencies.

Which Wines and Why?

Before offering any advice on the most suitable vintage to choose for rheumatic conditions, I should like to mention some recent statistics. These have established that in wine-growing regions where men are inclined to consume more wine than women, men are less affected by rheumatic diseases than women are. And Professor Mauriac has pointed out that gout sufferers are more numerous in countries where little wine is drunk.

Having said this, I certainly do not want to suggest that frequent recourse to the 'divine nectar' will provide protection against diseases of the joints, if not an actual cure. Nonetheless, apart from remedies prescribed in individual circumstances, it is true that, chosen with discernment and drunk in moderation, the juice of the vine occupies an honourable place in a clinically controlled diet. If the rheumatic illness presents with different symptoms, the choice of wine will likewise be different. I shall give the reasons for this later.

Inflammatory Arthritis

For rheumatic attacks accompanied by a rise in temperature, the use of red wines will be most appropriate, so long as your doctor approves. The arguments in favour of this type of vintage are based on centuries of experience, confirmed by the most recent scientific experiments. For acute pain in the joints accompanied by a sudden rise in temperature, the diet should include the wines of the Médoc region. Rich in pigments found in the pulp of the fruit, they possess genuine antibiotic properties. The dosage should be one or two glasses per meal.

Apart from these feverish attacks, because the patient's physical condition provides a favourable environment for the spread of inflammation and leaves him constantly at risk, it would be better to stay faithful to this type of red wine always. A half bottle a day will have an appropriate antibiotic effect.

Wine for Rheumatoid Arthritis

Arthritic symptoms affecting the joints may, at the outset, be quite temporary. Developing without sudden rises in temperature, this form of rheumatism is usually caused by toxic substances produced by the body, which affect the system and are characterised by a retention of urate or oxalate crystals. These must therefore be eliminated.

Accordingly, the choice of wine should tend towards the light white wines whose grapes have been treated with sulphur. The mineral ion sulphur exists naturally in the juice of the vine but its level is increased even further by the process of 'mitage'. This occurs during cellular oxidisation and through its centrifugal action this metalloid promotes the elimination of organic toxins. This property is confirmed through the results obtained from the sulphurated thermal cures taken by sufferers from chronic rheumatism.

People who have mild rheumatism should opt, depending on personal taste, either for the 'blancs de blancs' (white wine made with white grapes) of the Champagne region, which are alkalinising and diuretic, or for the wines of Alsace produced from the Sylvaner vinestock. The wines of Crépy are also recommended for the same reasons. As for the permitted dose, you should restrict yourself to two glasses per meal. However, if this type of arthritis sufferer has a tendancy to be overweight, he should avoid liqueur-like wines and those which, despite the respect due to them, have been in bottle for a certain number of years.

Wine for Osteoarthritis

Without wishing to think of wine in terms of a specific type of medication, its value to the osteoarthritis sufferer gives it a good claim to the title.

In one way, osteoarthritis can be regarded as a symptom of localised progressive degeneration of the joints. It indicates a deficiency in mineral salts, sodium, magnesium and manganese, affecting the ligaments and the bones.

Within the framework of the prescribed diet and medication, wine contributes the elements in which the body is deficient. Although this contribution may appear negligible in terms of quantity, its role is to provide catalytic agents which trigger off chemical reactions, aiding in the rebuilding of cells.

Before listing the vintages that are especially suitable for those with chronic arthritis, at the onset of this condition one could try the light wines of the Côtes du Rhône, Tavel or Lirac. Being rich in silicon salts, they help to maintain the balance of the calcium metabolism, thus ensuring the solidity and homogeneity of bone and joint tissue. However, because of their effect on kidney secretion, these vintages are not recommended for arthritics who suffer periodically from attacks of renal colic.

Among arthritics who also suffer from urinary sand,

without, however, acute attacks of kidney pains, the choice should be made from the rosé or white wines of Provence, like Cassis or Bandol, which contain magnesium salts. This element is a conveyor of phosphorus, which indirectly nourishes bone tissue in that its presence allows calcification. Moreover, because of their Mediterranean origin and their exposure to an exceptional amount of sunshine, these wines are rich in B complex vitamins and ascorbic acid. These products thus make a definite contribution in alleviating the pain associated with joint disorders.

The choice of wine will be different for those who have chronic arthritis. These patients should choose a vintage rich in manganese in its ionic form, such as is present in a natural state in grape juice. This catalysing agent works in the body in infinitesimal doses by aiding the breakdown of proteins, the metabolic slowing down of which promotes the formation of urates. In this way it represents a modifying element having a positive effect on the progress of arthritic joint disorders.

In France, which is so rich in varieties of wine, the soil of Corbières and in particular of Minervois is particularly rich in manganese oxide. The red wines of this region contain 1.5 mg to 2.5 mg per litre. They are therefore all suitable as table wines for the diet of arthritis sufferers.

This choice is not the only possible one. Apart from the manganese needed in arthritis, it is worth adding the mineral elements necessary for the remineralising of the bone tissue, in particular calcium phosphate. These will be found in the light, fruity red wines of the Côtes du Ventoux. The vines there are cultivated on a soil with a basis of cretaceous limestone, and the ancient ochre quarries in the area bear witness to the richness of this soil in iron oxides and manganese.

Whatever the choice of wines given above, the permitted dose should not exceed the equivalent of two glasses per meal.

WINE LIST

Vintages	Clinical Indications
Médoc	Acute rheumatism
Blanc de Blanc Crépy Sylvaner	Rheumatoid arthritis
Lirac Tavel Cassis Bandol	Mild osteoarthritis
Corbières Côtes du Ventoux Minervois	Chronic osteoarthritis

CHAPTER 5

WINE AND IMMUNISATION

Among various physiological functions that allow the body to live and, in some circumstances, to survive, one cannot neglect the importance of the one that enables it to respond with varying degrees of success to the pathogenic attacks of bacteria, viruses or parasites. This is its capacity for natural immunity from these agents.

Faced with microbic or viral attacks, the body immediately goes on the defensive in order, through its own resources, to annihilate the effects of foreign proteins whose action may cause illness. This healthy response may sometimes prove inadequate, and then needs to fall back on supplementary substances that will supply it with the means of defence it is momentarily lacking. Since the achievements of Jenner and Pasteur and the subsequent development and extension of antibiotic medicines, this battle against infection has enjoyed remarkable success. Preventative vaccines, serums, sulphamides and penicillins for curative purposes are now at our disposal, some as shields, others as offensive weapons.

In view of the widespread use of these therapeutic aids and taking into account the results obtained, one might wonder whether the juice of the vine still has a role to play. The answer is that, in this situation as in all those discussed above, wine has something to say.

Let us judge for ourselves!

A Brief History

In the days when the medicinal agents we have just mentioned were as yet unavailable to help fight infections of all kinds, physicians used, among other things, the bactericidal properties provided in the fermented juice of the vine. Without going back as far as Hippocrates and leaving aside practitioners of former times such as Celsus, Sydenham and many others, we might recall that Ambroise Paré made use of it by applying poultices of red wine to war wounds and burst ulcers. Furthermore, wine was taken as a protective medication during certain epidemics and proved an effective measure. I have given some examples in the chapter on the medicinal history of wine through the ages.

Without adding to the list of doctors and researchers who have recognised the positive action of wine in treating infectious diseases and their after-effects, one can say that this beverage provides immunisation which is both preventative and curative against pathogenic germs and viral toxins. Moreover, following serious bacterial infections, when these are treated with classic antibiotics, massive doses extended over too long a period can lead to a state of fatigue which further complicates the fatigue resulting from the illness itself. In such cases wine, through certain of its components, acts as a physical and mental stimulant and helps to restore the disturbed metabolism to working order. I shall be returning to this latter property during the next chapter.

The Antibiotic Elements in Wine

Evidence of the immunising property of wine, and more particularly that of red wines, was confirmed by the experimental research of Professor J. Masquelier and his colleagues, J. Michaud and H. Jensen. Through the processes of fermentation and ageing, the natural chemical transformations taking place in this beverage lead to the formation of oenidol, which comes from the anthocyanins, coloured pigments from the skin of the grape. Their antibiotic value depends on their quality and abundance. Although young wines have only a negligible effect on the action of microbes, vintages which have been in the bottle for several years (between 7 and 15 years) develop a more obvious bactericidal action.

Two Canadian experts, Doctors Spier and Konowalchick, have also demonstrated that red wine, rich in tannoid products, attacks certain viruses, such as those responsible for herpes and poliomyelitis. The proteins that make up the chemical structure of these elements, on becoming infectious, combine with the tannin of the grape juice and thus lose their harmfulness.

To a lesser degree the white wines, through the leucoanthocyans they contain, exercise a vitamin P action which gives them an antibiotic effect. Apart from the gastronomic tradition that associates oysters with white wine, one can see it as an instinctive safeguard against the infectious bacteria of this type of shellfish.

Strawberries in Wine

This delicious summer dessert is not available to everyone because of the fruit's potentially allergic effects in the form of hives.

In order not to deprive these hypersensitive people of a simple gastronomic delight, Doctor Weisseimbach advises them to soak the fruit for a quarter of an hour in a bowl of red wine before eating them. In this way they can satisfy their gourmet appetite without suffering the irritating consequences.

Several theories have been proposed to explain the anti-allergic action of fermented grape juice and more especially that of red wines, which are rich in tannin. In the opinion of these researchers, this phenomenon has nothing to do with the antibiotic properties of these wines. To understand how they work, we should turn to the writings of J. Masquelier on the role of the pyocyanidins of wine. Through their vitamin P action these elements control the permeability of the arterial walls. In allergy sufferers, the increase in degree of an enzyme, histadin (an amino-acid made up of proteins) transforms it into histamine which dilates the walls of the capillaries. The alteration in the permeability of the blood vessels thus promotes the passage of blood serum which spreads into the surrounding tissues forming local or generalised swellings. According to Dr Masquelier, red wine combats this excess production of histamine, which is responsible for allergic reactions.

Wine and Toxins

Without leaving the field of the protective action of wine against microbic or viral toxins, we should add a word on its role in relation to toxic products other than foreign proteins.

The ancient Roman naturalist Pliny the Elder regarded the juice of the vine as an antidote to poison, not only in cases of snake-bite but also in treating the unfortunate consequences of eating poisonous mushrooms. Since his time, many clinicians have recommended this beverage as a defensive agent against intoxicating medicines. In spite of these assertions, many worthy people, inspired by the very best intentions, have roundly declared that the 'divine nectar' is in itself a poison. Like any extreme opinion, it can only give rise to scepticism.

The Choice of Wine

In order to deal with the different situations described in the preceding paragraphs, we must take three factors into account when choosing our wine: its colour, its age, and its composition. In these circumstances, one should give preference to red wines which have been at least five years in the bottle, are rich in oenotannins, in vitamins C and P and contain manganese. Since this type of wine is predominant in wine production, we must narrow the field according to the cause and nature of the disease. If the wine is chosen to take account of the existing clinical symptoms and the stage of the illness, it will act as preventative medication, if not as a medicinal supplement to the remedies prescribed.

DURING BACTERIAL OR VIRAL ATTACKS

In this era of antibiotics that are natural or chemically based, the treatment of infectious disease has had, and is still having, remarkable success. Sometimes there are setbacks, too. However, taken in excess or misused, such medication leaves the body in a state of fatigue and less resistant to future attacks.

To lessen these drawbacks and to help the body in its fight, it is beneficial to complement the prescribed medication by taking Médoc wines, or even the wines of St Estephe or Listrac, as table wines. Coming from vine varieties grown on a soil rich in ferrous oxide and organic phosphorus, these elements are also found in the fermented juice of the vine. For the invalid they have a tonic and restorative factor which is indispensable during feverish attacks. But their importance is increased by the fact that they contain oenotannins which give them antibiotic properties.

You can also choose from the red wines of Beaujolais, which are equally rich in oenidol. A half bottle of one or other of these wines, divided between the two main meals, meets the needs of the patient and supplies him with the necessary medicinal supplement.

During winter epidemics these same wines should also be used as long as the danger of contagion persists. Without having regular recourse to the more distinguished 'châteaux' wines, better Côtes de Bordeaux reds are also quite acceptable and are rich in mineral salts.

DURING CONVALESCENCE

The after-effects of a bacterial or viral attack can be a state of fatigue that may go as far as mental depression. Such attacks weaken the body and this can trigger off a relapse. Here wine is a valuable medicine. In this final stage of the illness your first choice should be the red wines of Burgundy, such as the various wines of the Côte de Nuits, which are rich in mineral and ferrous salts. They supply the body that has been weakened by illness with elements containing restorative properties. But in spite of these qualities, they are not recommended for those suffering from high blood pressure, for the obese or those suffering from gout. The latter should turn to the red wines of Beaujolais, which are generous and tonic, uplifting and make good any mineral deficiencies. In both cases, half a bottle a day is an effective and reasonable dose.

Still with the same aim of restoring organic and functional order, never forget the beneficial effects of extra-dry Champagne, due to its natural phosphorus content. Its glucose and fructose content also helps to restore energy. Finally, its high sulphuric ion content gives it cleansing and purgative properties which encourage the elimination of toxins accumulated during the illness.

Convalescents will find it beneficial to follow an eight-day cure taking daily and in little sips (*noblesse oblige*) the equivalent of two glasses of a good extra-dry or dry Champagne during the quarter of an hour preceding a meal.

AND FOR ALLERGICS

As this sufferer has much in common with arthritics, to alleviate the symptoms he should turn to the properties of manganese. A basic remedy in the treatment of this condition, it acts as a catalytic agent. Like the sufferer from chronic rheumatism, the allergy sufferer should supplement his diet with the wines of Corbières, Minervois and Côtes de Ventoux. I have given the reasons for this in the chapter on the role of wine in joint disorders.

WINE LIST

Vintages	Clinical Indications
Beaujolais Listrac Médoc St-Estephe	Bacterial illnesses
Côtes de Bordeaux (premières)	Preventing influenza attacks
Côtes de Nuits Champagne (extra-dry or dry)	Convalescence
Corbières Côtes du Ventoux Minervois	Allergies

CHAPTER 6

WINE AND THE METABOLISM

To feed a glowing fire, which in return supplies heat and contributes to the maintenance of life, we need a fuel able to fulfil this function. The choice and volume of calorie supply depend on needs. However, this operation ends in the production of waste which must be eliminated to avoid choking the fire and causing it to function less efficiently.

I chose this metaphor to give an idea of the important function of the metabolism, since it is obvious that quite a number of biochemical factors come into play where the human body is concerned. Among these factors, wine plays a part in many different ways in all kinds of body functions.

At the heart of all living matter, the elements produced to allow it to exist and expend energy undergo a series of chemical transformations. But these processes should not lead to an imbalance in the system and to symptoms of illness, resulting from insufficient intracellular oxygenation. If this happens, there will be a retention of wastes that will lodge in the organ tissues.

Imperfectly metabolised, these products, depending on the individual case or temperament, will be lipids in obesity, protids in uricaemia, gout or kidney stones, or glucids in diabetes. For each of these conditions, advice on the appropriate wines will be given at the end of this chapter.

Without going further into biological details, we can say that these metabolic changes depend, by and large, either on a slowing down in the process or on its acceleration—in other words, on a lack of balance between what is supplied and what is discarded as waste.

In an overall therapy, apart from a diet adapted to each of these conditions, it is important to consider other intervening factors: the catalytic action of the vitamins and that of the endocrine glands whose enzyme products contribute to slowing down or accelerating (depending on the case) the processes of chemical transformation of the nutriments. In the forefront of this process is the liver. A satisfactory functioning of the metabolic complex guarantees the stability of an acid-base equilibrium, tending rather towards alkalinity, and helps with the elimination of waste products.

Wine and Acid-base Equilibrium

A satisfactory state of health and resistance to disease both depend on the balance between the alkalinity of the body's internal organs and their acidity, while trying to keep the pH* of the blood in a state of relative alkalinity. According to some dieticians, this aim is achieved by keeping to a diet containing predominantly vegetarian and dairy products. However, the addition of wine to the daily menu leads to the same result. In fact, among its components we can count organic acids (lactic, tartaric, citric, malic, and so on) acting in infinitesimal doses through their catalytic action and contributing, after chemical conversion, to the formation of alkaline carbonates. These elements act on the oxidising mechanism, so maintaining the level of alkalinity. The acid-base equilibrium is thus achieved and maintained.

* pH = potential hydrogen, a coefficient characterising the acidity or alkalinity of a medium.

Protids, Glucids and Lipids

The action of wine goes further than this initial effect. In the metabolic process, constructive elements are supplied to the system and after utilisation the waste matter is expelled. Because of the vitamins it contains, wine plays a useful role in getting this process moving and ensuring a balance between what is supplied and what needs to be eliminated.

The metabolism of proteins is partly due to the presence of riboflavin (vitamin B2) which accelerates their conversion, preventing the formation of urea.

As for the glucids, the mechanism that effects their combustion is activated by the presence of other vitamins of the B complex, thiamin and riboflavin, already mentioned above. These elements help in their assimilation and indirectly regulate their conversion into calories.

The fats, for their part, are altered by the action of meso-inositol (vitamin I), present in grape juice. Doctor Lucia, Director of Medical Research at the American Wine Office, has pointed out in this connection that if wine is drunk on a regular basis, but only at the end of a meal, as an aid to digestion, it is possible to reduce the daily food intake, resulting in a weight loss of up to 1,600 grammes per week. And Professor Fiessinger has noted that habitual wine drinkers are often thin and lean.

The Liver and the Other Glands

In the process of metabolism, the liver is particularly active in converting glucids supplied by wine alcohol, due to an oxidising enzyme which converts alcoholic molecules into water and carbonic gas. This conversion, particularly noticeable with red wines, generates heat, a process which is increased if sugar is added to the beverage. This supply of calories has a particular role with elderly people or with those who feel the need for a restorative after strenuous physical exercise. However, this operation depends on a healthy liver and the dose must not exceed the liver's oxidising capacity.

In another chemical process, the glycerol in the wine combines with organic phosphates to form glycerophosphates which tone up the nervous system and reduce the need for lipids and glucids.

Independently of the liver, other endocrine glands, activated in their turn by the consumption of wine during meals, play a part in the chemical conversion of the nutriments ingested. Wine promotes the secretion of pancreatic juice, rich in lipase, an enzyme which metabolises fats.

The thyroid is affected by the action of certain components of the fermented juice of the vine, in particular by wine coming from vines cultivated in a micro-climate rich in iodine, as is the case for the wines of the Mediterranean Languedoc and Provence. According to Loeper, this thyroid activity accelerates the destruction of wastes resulting from the assimilation and conversion processes.

Wine and Metabolic Imbalances

We shall not dwell on the causes of metabolic changes, nor on wine's role in the matter, since these have been discussed at length in the author's book, *Notre Vin Quotidien*. Here we shall merely mention some factors and recommend appropriate wines.

ACIDOSIS

The excessive production of acids in the internal organs is due to a defective conversion of the amino-acids supplied to the body by the proteins in food. Apart from medical and dietary treatment, the sufferer from acidosis should make his choice of table wine from the wines of Nivernais, Pouilly or Sancerre, which are rich in alkaline carbonates and in tartrates.

MINERAL DIFICIENCY

Body losses in mineral salts, if these are compounds of calcium, require a wine diet rich in red wines, low in alcohol but containing elements which will make up the deficiencies in such cases. The sufferer should opt for the wines of the Premières Côtes de Bordeaux, coming from vines cultivated on a soil of siliceous and chalky clay type. The Beaujolais wines, from a soil rich in mineral salts, are also suitable. On the other hand, if the mineral deficiencies are phosphatic salts, causing physical fatigue and mental depression, the Champagne wines are very suitable. Their vines flourish on a soil rich in phosphoric acid. Not only that, they have the added bonus of ascorbic acid (vitamin C). The most noble of all, an extra-dry variety, should be chosen and two glasses may be taken as an apéritif.

URICAEMIA

An excess of uric or oxalic salt in the blood or the internal organs can lead to the formation of urinary sand, or gout. Those who suffer from this condition should select wines rich in organic acids and containing diuretic properties; these promote alkalinity in the body fluids and stimulate the flow of kidney secretion, thus removing urate or oxalate wastes in the urine.

Uricaemia sufferers should choose dry white wines of the Loire Valley, such as Muscadet or Gros Plan, which are rich in potassium and therefore diuretic, or else the Sancerre wines, which contain tartrates and organic acids, and are therefore alkalinising.

DIABETES

Without going into the causes and symptoms of this type of metabolic imbalance, we should emphasise the importance of including vitamins of the B complex in the diet of the diabetic, especially thiamin and pantothenic acid. These catalytic agents replace pancreatic enzymes which are insufficient or even absent. Their presence helps the body to metabolise blood sugars, a process that is boosted even more by the presence in wine of a metallic ion, chromium (at the rate of 450 mg per litre). This substance activates insulin, enabling it to process the glucose that has been ingested. What is more, through its fructose content wine, the true 'bread of the diabetic', constitutes a 'storage' food, compensating for the restrictions on starchy foods. Finally, for diabetics who are overweight, this beverage, through its glycerol content, promotes the secretion of pancreatic lipases which metabolise fats.

Wine included as part of the daily menu should, however, be selected to suit the physiological restrictions imposed by this type of metabolic disorder. The diabetic should therefore abstain from mellow or liqueur-like wines. On the other hand, he can take red Bordeaux wines with his meals, which are light and low in alcohol, or Alsatian wines such as Riesling or Sylvaner.

The equivalent of half a bottle a day, divided between the two main meals, is a suitable dose.

GOUT

Bearing in mind Professor Mauriac's observation that there are few gout sufferers in wine-growing regions, one might add that the fermented juice of the vine has a role to play in combating this condition, when it is chosen wisely and drunk at the right time.

During an acute attack of gout, the rule is to go on a water diet and help the functioning of the kidneys by drinking mineral waters such as Evian or Vittel. But apart from these crises, gout sufferers, who are actually arthritics, should supplement their diet with light, dry, white wines which have alkalinising and diuretic properties. The Savoy vineyards offer a whole range of Crépy or Seyssel wines.

OBESITY

This condition is often brought about by errors in diet or health care, or may be the result of metabolic changes affecting the lipids and blood sugars, traceable to the glands. The fats supplied to the body through food are only partially converted and eliminated. They are retained in the organs or in the subcutaneous cell tissue, creating in the first case the folds of fat called 'exogenous' and in the second retentions of serum forming 'cellulite'.

Leaving the doctor to work out a diet and decide on the appropriate treatment, we shall only deal here with the wine aspect of the problem.

In cases of what is known as 'exogenous' obesity, the problem for the medical wine waiter is how to encourage the metabolism of fats and, in the case of cellulite, to eliminate excess serum.

In both cases, wines rich in alcohol and sugar should be avoided, such as apéritifs (except for extra-dry Champagne), digestifs, liqueur-type wines, lemonades, and manufactured fizzy drinks. Beer should be light and with an alcohol content not exceeding four degrees.

For people who have a tendency to become overweight, a carefully chosen wine, taken preferably towards the end of the meal, will promote digestion and help the absorption of the food. There is no need to remind you yet again that a meal washed down with water is drowned by that insipid beverage whose sole function is to quench thirst. On the other hand, the presence of meso-inositol in grape juice promotes the conversion of fatty foods. Finally, wine plays a role in stimulating the glandular secretions by acting on the liver, pituitary and thyroid glands.

People who are obese should opt for young red wines of 8 to 11 per cent alcoholic strength, but low in sugars. According to individual taste, you should choose either Bordeaux or Beaujolais-Villages wines. The permitted dose should not exceed one to two glasses, to be taken towards the end of the meal.

On the other hand, in cases of retention of serum in the subcutaneous cell tissues, as happens in the build-up of cellulite, one's preference should be for dry white wines with diuretic properties, such as Muscadet or Gros Plan. The reasons for such a choice were given in the chapter on the relationship between wine and the eliminatory functions.

WINE LIST

Vintages	Clinical Indications
Pouilly Sancerre	Acidosis and Uricaemia
Côtes de Bordeaux Beaujolais Champagne (extra-dry) Saint-Croix de Moum Saumur	Mineral deficiency
Bordeaux (red) Riesling Sylvaner Traminer	Diabetes and Obesity
Crépy Seyssel	Gout
Gros-Plan Muscadet	Cellulite

CHAPTER 7
WINE AND THE PSYCHE

It is human nature to fret. Over the years, the anxiety that we brought with us into the world has increased and worsened to match the rate of progress which a more and more automated and frenzied civilisation has so lavishly heaped upon us. It is no wonder that a characteristic of modern society should be this need to shut ourselves off by any means and so put off having to face up to our immediate problems; anything to avoid the moment when society dictates that we should relax and have nothing to do. Even as long ago as the seventeenth century Pascal noted, 'the only thing that consoles us for our miseries is amusement.'

The use of tranquillisers and drugs that has become so widespread today, and the refusal to recognise the habit as an illness, are reflections of this need to escape from ourselves. All we get out of it is a hangover and the knowledge that we are heading for physical, moral and mental degeneration.

Anti-alcohol campaigns, waged under the banner of healthy living, have also attacked wine. This movement, generated in a fervour of spartan puritanism, has contributed to the trend for using narcotics of all kinds, by trying to deny this human need for 'recreation'.

Throughout human history, and in every part of the world, people have always searched for a relief from their anxieties. In our moderate regions, why forbid them to turn for help to a noble beverage, so long as they drink it wisely, rather than deprive them of the benefits it can bring to their mental well-being?

For the benefit of wine's detractors, I shall devote the final chapter of Part Two to the relationship between wine and the brain centres—that is, the seat of the mind and the emotions. They do say, after all, that 'wine goes to the head'.

Having discussed wine's association with the main functions of the body, let us end by considering its influence on the psyche. Without defending its effect on the behaviour of people who abuse it by drinking more than they can hold, I shall therefore remain silent on the symptoms associated with drunkenness, even if it is regarded as 'sacred'.

My aim here is to throw light on the pleasant effects of the 'divine nectar' in the mental sphere, when it is chosen for its quality and treated wisely and sensibly.

All those qualities, both intellectual and sensory, that confer nobility on the human being are influenced by wine. The brain responds to its appeal by awakening its creative and emotional faculties, both as instigator and controller.

If it goes beyond a certain level of emotional tension, this heightened feeling may well cause a sensation of physical pain that may lead to a temporary or permanent state of agitation and anxiety. If this distress exceeds a certain tolerance threshold, it then requires the help of psychologists, if not psychiatrists who will administer tranquillisers which, however, are toxic. Rather than reaching this point, it is wiser to turn to a natural mood enhancer, the fermented juice of the vine. As the seventeenth-century theologian and friend of Pascal, Maître de Sacy, so aptly remarked, 'What is life for those who lack wine? It was created for the gaiety of mankind.'

Mental Harmony

Professor Fiessinger who, in his time, taught a whole generation of medical students, pointed out in his masterly lectures that 'wine maintains a correct balance between the mental outlook and the play of feelings.'

This quality, which proves the influence of the physical on the mental and vice versa, can be explained at a physiological level. In fact, the happy blend of sensory stimuli aroused by the colour, bouquet and aroma of a good quality vintage is transmitted by the pyramidal nervous pathway to the cerebral cortex and pleasantly titillates the emotional centres of the brain. The response is apparent in a feeling of calmness which is a valuable aid to thinking. As a result, one's judgement is sharpened, one becomes kinder, the spirit blossoms and worries are temporarily dispelled. From an intelligent communion with wine one derives a natural well-being which helps one cope better with the hazards of daily life. Is this not a kind of psychotherapy?

Hippocrates accused melancholy or 'black humour' of being the root cause of a number of illnesses. The treatment of this psychological condition included, among other remedies, the pursuit of cheerfulness, a state of mind which, according to the Master of Cos, dilates the passages of the spleen. Since those far-off times, humanity's needs in this respect have scarcely changed at all.

A Boost to the Morale

If the juice of the vine gives mental harmony to anyone who is in good health, the addition of wine to raise the spirits is equally desirable in the diet of many invalids.* It can only prove beneficial to make use of this medicinal

* See *Wine is the Best Medicine*, Dr E. Maury, Souvenir Press.

supplement, chosen to suit the individual case. To give just one example, certain vintages, such as the wines of Champagne, through their alcohol and phosphate content provide a nerve tonic which will give a boost to jaded spirits. A more modest wine, but just as effective in its action on the central nervous system, whether following an emotional shock or a serious illness, Blanquette de Limoux can also act as a buoy which is always pleasant to hang on to.

A Creative Factor

One of the traits that ennobles humanity is our creative faculty. Wine drinking, which helps achieve a good physiological balance, guaranteeing in its turn a good mental balance, leads to creative work, however modest it might be. The human body is not based solely on the mechanistic principles so dear to materialists. It is the seat of a mind that controls the whole. Just as the juice of the vine, through its chemical components, can boost a flagging system as a medicinal auxiliary, so at the same time it acts through its own soul on the creative genius of the human being. This spiritual contribution, which has been sensed by dreamers and sung of by many poets, stimulates the mental faculties by keeping the mind alert, and represents another factor in recovery. To cite just a single example, but one of some importance, let us refer once more to the good Master François Rabelais, doctor of medicine at the Faculty of Montpellier and a great enthusiast of the 'divine nectar', who urged us to abstract its 'essential substance'. The key to the Wisdom hidden deep in the bottle, we may extract its philosophical teaching by intelligent intercourse with its contents. In his capacity as a doctor, he surely meant to suggest, through this counsel, that beyond Wisdom we might also rediscover Health there, in the widest sense of the word. For this genuine optimist, the juice of the vine clarifies the mind and the understanding, allays anger, banishes sadness, gives joy and light-heartedness.

In the mind of this native of Touraine, steeped in the vintages of his native soil, human wisdom can be summed up in one word: 'DRINK', but using this word in its widest sense. If the term covers the physiological need nobly to quench a legitimate thirst, it presupposes for the moralist and philosopher the alleviation of the spiritual longings slumbering in the hearts of all decent folk.

Since we are looking at the influence of wine on our creative powers, we cannot ignore the inhabitants of the gentle Loire countryside, rich in quality vintages. This was the home of the sixteenth-century poets of the 'Pleiade' group led by Pierre de Ronsard, whose verses impart the savour of the wines of Anjou. And in sampling the sonnets of Ronsard, we rediscover the sweet and heady flavour of the vintages produced on the banks of that majestic river. In leafing through the pages of the *Regrets* of Joachim du Bellay, another member of the 'Pleiade', we feel, with the poet, nostalgia for the Angevin wines which the bouquet of their Italian counterparts cannot dispel.

Still in the field of literary creativity, if we turn to the south-west we can steep ourselves in the passionate soul of the wines of Cahors which revive memories of the poems of Clément Marot (1496–1544), who sang the praises of that 'strong and full-flavoured liquor'.

And what can one say of the authors who spent their lives in the Bordeaux region? Michel de Montaigne, sixteenth-century moralist and himself a wine-grower, recalled in his *Essays* the need for wisdom based on tolerance and level-headedness, conduct dictated, very likely, by friendly communion with the wines of Médoc. As for Montesquieu, in his works we find the solid framework which is characteristic of Graves and Pomerol wines.

We have barely touched on the many poets and prose writers born and bred in wine-growing regions; we cannot name every one, but they all have one thing in common: according to where they grew up, their works bear the stamp of the wines of their native region. Who was better able than Colette, the Burgundian, with her flair and sensitivity, to understand the soul hidden in the juice of the vine and the lesson it gave its drinkers? 'I am proud,' she wrote, 'to have grown up, matured and aged on intimate terms with wine; having been familiar with it since childhood, one loses the spirit of intemperance and gluttony; one acquires, one forms one's personal taste.'

This spirit of creativity, drawn from the 'divine nectar', is evidence of an art of living and a joy in living. If it is sometimes hidden, it will always surface in those millions of bubbles that rise from a glass of Champagne. It took a man dedicated to God, Dom Pierre Pérignon, cellarer of the Abbey of Hautvillers in the Marne district, inspired by the pagan influence of Bacchus, to blend the vintages of different varieties of vine. By this act of creation was born a beverage of incomparable quality, which can only be produced in the soil of Champagne. It does not need us to exalt its virtues and describe how it affects the emotional centres of the brain by arousing the noble functions of the spirit. For E. T. A. Hoffmann, that teller of fairy-tales, Champagne was the 'poetic wine'. As for its influence on female beauty, I refer you to the opinion of just one of them, who was well versed in the matter, Madame de Pompadour. And for the visionary this wine is a synthesis of 'the brilliant image of the French'. The soul that haunts this beverage reflects, even beyond the country that gave it birth, that of a whole people.

It is up to them to understand and preserve it.

PART THREE
WINE AND THE TEMPERAMENTS

'Wine taken in moderation is a second life; if you take it moderately, you will be sober.'

Sacy, *L'Ecclesiastique*, XXXXI

This book, dedicated to Hippocrates, has dealt with wine from the point of view of our physiological or psychological reactions to it. Still in the same vein and keeping in mind the Doctrine of the Master of Cos, I thought it might be interesting to propose a hypothesis, which might offer a more original and wide-ranging concept of wine. This is in fact only my own theory.

Throughout this book, the product of the grape has been treated as a living being, with a personality of its own and hence possessing both a body and a soul. However, on reflection, it struck me that from this standpoint there should be a final element, which would make up its expression and synthesis. It would unite, in a single entity, the material being, of physical nature, and the spiritual being, of more subtle character. In another way, we can find in ourselves the same biological synthesis that we can find in what we drink. Here I refer to that reality, concerning both the physical and the mental, which Hippocrates described in his time by the general term of 'temperament'.

The Greek physician's study of the whole human being led him to define four types, and it is on this number of four that we should base our wider study of the product of the vine.

I have therefore tried, in the pages that follow, to trace the same phenomenon in wine and hence to apply it to what one can also find in any living and thinking individual. It goes without saying that this attempt is no more than a theory which may seem outrageous, but all the same, it would have been wrong to keep it to myself.

CHAPTER 1

THE HIPPOCRATIC CONCEPT

A correct understanding of the terminology will help to make my meaning clear. Plato himself said that 'knowledge of words leads to the knowledge of things'. Although the term 'temperament' has different connotations in modern parlance from that given it in Hippocratic medical doctrine, it does have a precise meaning, based on a cosmic view of the human being.

What was the reasoning followed by its author?

Homo sapiens, emerging by successive stages from his primitive animal state, began to observe the natural phenomena he witnessed daily, and he tried to classify them. What he had realised was that the manifestations of nature, of whatever order, followed periodic cycles which recur regularly and in the final analysis take on a rhythm based on the number FOUR.

He was convinced of the truth of this discovery by the existence of the four cosmic elements, the four seasons of the year, the four ages of life, the four cardinal points. This list, including other natural phenomena, could be extended to infinity and includes, in turn, the biological phenomena affecting the human being. Hippocrates then applied this 'quaternary' (or fourfold) concept to man as a whole to obtain more complete knowledge, both physiological and pathological. He identified four essential functions in the body: nutrition, breathing, the antitoxic functions (what we call metabolism) and excretion. Each of these functions is performed by means of different body liquids which he called the four 'Humours': blood, lymph or phlegm, bile and black bile.

Each of these, according to its predominance over the others, contributes to the formation of a specific 'Temperament' of which there are again four: sanguine, nervous, lymphatic (or phlegmatic) and melancholy. Their reciprocal balance guarantees the continuance of life and maintenance of physical and mental health.

From the modern scientific viewpoint the Hippocratic doctrine, through its apparent simplicity, appears outdated. However, the anatomical elements involved still exist in the body, and their respective functions have not altered at all since the time of the 83rd Olympiad. It is really just their names that have changed, and we now know more about how they work and what can go wrong.

The fact still remains that blood provides food, that bile activates digestive metabolic functions, that lymph makes the organs supple and that black bile, an excess of which contributes to the formation of stones, still plays a supporting role for the other humours. Even now, it would be impossible to imagine a body in which one or other of these humours was lacking.

At certain times in one's life, one of them is dominant throughout the system and then confers on the individual a typological, physiological and psychological aspect that constitutes what Hippocrates defined as being the 'Temperament' (or single dominant characteristic) peculiar to that person. At the present time, a number of practitioners have taken up this Hippocratic concept again, and are adapting it as a holistic approach to the individual. Its aspects have been defined under the more general heading of 'biological terrain'.

Among these contemporary researchers, we could cite J. Menetrier and his colleagues, whose work, in turn, has enabled us to distinguish four different types of 'terrain' or 'condition'. These researches and their results have led to the use of trace elements in medical treatment. It is worth pointing out that these infinitesimal amounts are found in wine, which could partly explain the medicinal action of that beverage.

After reading the foregoing, you may well wonder what place wine occupies in all this.

CHAPTER 2

THE 'QUATERNARY' OF THE GRAPE

The theory proposed in these pages might seem, to any rational and Cartesian mind, to have emanated from an imagination heightened by an abuse of Bacchic libations. But if one looks at it objectively, this research throws light on mysteries that puzzle any questioning mind, as well as responding to our need to find a satisfactory explanation for the phenomena of life.

When looking at a bunch of grapes, why shouldn't we take note of any new evidence of this 'quaternary' which, as well as revealing a truth, also leads to a broader understanding of natural phenomena?

If we look at it just from the 'anatomical' point of view, we cannot help seeing that the fruit of the vine which will later yield its juice is composed of four parts: the stalk, the outer skin, the pulp and the seeds. This whole, in its coherence and harmony, resembles a true living organism.

On the other hand, from the biological angle we can see that the grapes pass through four distinct stages of development. They go from the state which one could term 'foetal' to their final use that we know so well, passing through the transformation of the flower into fruit (setting), the beginning of maturation (ripening) and finally full maturation. Just like all other manifestations of life, this progress towards the final goal can be compared to that of the four main periods of human existence: childhood, adolescence, adulthood and old age.

To return to the vine, its fruiting cycle is accomplished

in harmony with the four seasons of the year. It begins during the winter period of preparation, followed by the blossoming of spring, succeeded by summer ripening to end in the sacrifice of the autumn grape harvest. This process also requires the participation of the four cosmic elements: the earth of the native soil that nourishes, the fire of the sun that warms, the water from the skies that swells the fruit and finally the air of the surrounding micro-climate which supplies oxygen. After reading this, how can one fail to see that this 'quaternary' permeates the plant that was created for our delight? What is more, might we not find it at work again, at the very heart of its product, wine?

CHAPTER 3

THE 'QUATERNARY' IN THE BOTTLE

This theory, aimed at defining the place of the number FOUR in relation to the juice of the vine, gains further support from a new idea—that there is a harmony between the contents of the bottle and the cosmic elements which have helped to create it. Like the preceding example, this is merely a point of view, of interest only in that it may satisfy our very natural curiosity by following a particular line of inquiry.

Aside from any purely oenological consideration, we can still see that, from the physical point of view, such as the colour and consistency of the liquid, the product of the vine can be divided into four categories each with its own intrinsic quality: the red wines, the white wines, the rosé wines and the liqueur-type wines. Some readers may be surprised to find the latter figuring in a separate category. My answer would be that the very qualities of these wines distinguish them from their fellows, if only by their colour, russet or golden according to the vintages, their alcohol content and the degree of concentration of the elements they contain. And while we are on the subject of these wines, we might make another point that again proves the significance of the number four. These wines can in fact only be produced from four different varieties of vine, muscat, grenache, malvoisie and maccabeo. It follows that they deserve to have a category distinct from the others, which adds support to this theory that the 'quaternary' has a definite place in our view of wine.

Pushing on in the same vein as we continue our search

for new examples, we shall find that in their respective qualities elements of the cosmos are echoed in the fermented product of the vine.

We could therefore liken red wine to the element of FIRE, dispenser of heat, white wine to the element of WATER, generator of humidity, rosé wine to the element AIR, the substance that purifies and oxygenates, and finally, liqueur-like wines to the element of EARTH, symbol of stability and firmness.

Categorising wines in this way, by linking similarities of colour and characteristic between a wine and its cosmic counterpart, however arbitrary it may seem, is nevertheless based on certain material facts. If we consider the physical properties of grape juice, which give each category of wine its individuality, we can see how one or the other of the cosmic elements might provide a further link between what one might call the 'temperament' of the wines and the needs of the individual.

To illustrate this theory, let's look at some examples.

Through their respective properties, the red wines primarily affect the circulation; the white wines, by stimulating the work of the kidneys, increase urination; the rosé wines cleanse the system by speeding up the metabolism. Finally, the liqueur-like wines, rich in restorative elements, strengthen the anatomical structure.

In the spirit of the Hippocratic concept as it applies to the whole human being, and to conclude this research, we can identify one last link—between the specific characteristics that distinguish the four different categories of wines and the 'temperaments' that dominate the human mind and body according to its 'humours', as taught in the Doctrine of the Quaternary.

CHAPTER 4

THE 'QUATERNARY' IN THE HUMOURS AND IN WINE

Without embarking on a psychological study, which would go beyond the scope of this book, it must be said that, by nature and in our likes and dislikes, we humans struggle to escape from the monotony of uniformity. We assert our preferences, let our dislikes be known. In general this also applies to our feelings about wine.

Although the great majority of people always enjoy drinking wine, nevertheless there are some who do not like it. They may have been introduced to it in the wrong way, or their choice of wine may clash with their biological personality and their temperament. I shall come back to this matter a little later. As for the rest of us, especially in the wine-growing regions and irrespective of what we eat, we study the wine list with care before selecting the vintage that will best complement our meal. Whether we opt for red or white, we will unconsciously give preference to the vintage that corresponds to our own particular needs.

In pursuit of our thesis proving this correlation between the physical expressions of the 'quaternary' and the different 'humours', we might wonder whether our choice of wine is influenced by the dominant humour of our temperament, in the Hippocratic sense of the term. We can then envisage a symbolic agreement between the wine a person chooses and his own temperament. In a word, is there a connection between the 'terrain' of the individual and that of the wine he or she chooses?

In answering this question I must provide short descriptions both typological and psychological, of each of the four individual temperaments, with their respective 'dominant'. I shall then try to match up the essential traits of each with their wine counterparts which resemble them in their qualities and intrinsic properties.

Again, this is only a hypothesis, if not a flight of fancy, but it is worth attempting.

The Sanguine Temperament

The dominants belonging to this physiological type are related to two functions: breathing and circulation. The individual in this category of humour, more than any other, has a need for air and movement to activate the blood flow.

From the typological point of view, the sanguine type is of average size, and stocky. He has a broad face, red cheeks, lively, laughing eyes. His skin is warm, his movements supple; he is given to large and frequent gesticulations.

Psychologically he is an enthusiast, an optimist, sometimes quick-tempered, but nevertheless fond of good living. He is a prime example of the extrovert type.

His health prospects will be affected by the bad eating habits arising from his taste for the good life, but above all by a deficiency or lack of the elements indispensable to his good humoral balance. His sedentary way of life combined with a lack of fresh air will eventually lead to high blood pressure and obesity. These same conditions can in their turn cause a poisoning of the system, because proteins are not properly digested and so lead to the formation of urates and oxalates and, in consequence, rheumatism, gout or urinary sand. Apart from changing to a healthy lifestyle and a diet geared to suit his individual biological terrain, where wine is concerned the 'sanguine' type should avoid old or liqueur-like wines, which are too heavy for his temperament.

He should instead choose from the dry white wines, which are light and amusing, in particular those that best symbolise the element of AIR, the dominant of this humoral type. He will find the wine that suits him best in the vintages of the Champagne region, extra-dry, semi-sparkling and aerated. Champagne, which brings joy and lightens the heart, corresponds to the psyche of our 'sanguine' type. What is more, thanks to its components, this wine guarantees a good physiological balance for this type of temperament by its effect on the heart, arteries and kidneys.

The Nervous Temperament

The dominant of this humoral type is related to the functions of elimination, which are either sluggish or over-active. Again we can see how this is reflected in the typology of the individual and his psyche, and from these features can understand his health problems.

The 'nervous' type is recognisable by his triangular face and his broad, high forehead. His eyes are mobile and expressive, his skin dry, pale and cold.

In his behaviour he betrays by word and gesture a certain reserve due to his lack of assurance. To compensate for this weakness, of which he is aware, he often resorts to cunning, putting forward his ideas tentatively until he is sure of his ground, when he states his case clearly and firmly.

From the physiological point of view, sluggishness or disturbances of the excretory functions tend to lead to sclerosis affecting the tissues of the arteries and the organs, a process that could well cause premature ageing. The cosmic element of the 'nervous' type is symbolised by the EARTH. He has its solidity, reliability and superficial coldness, but if one digs deeper, one discovers his warmth. We find some of these traits in historical characters who can serve as illustration of the typological description given above. We can cite, for example, Montaigne, Montesquieu and, nearer to our own time, François Mauriac, all three natives of the Bordeaux region. This circumstance naturally leads one to equate this type of humour with the red wines of their native country, Médoc, St-Emilion or Pomérol.

These Gironde vintages, produced from a gravelly soil, are suitable for the 'nervous' type, who is timid and cold, through their gently stimulating and heat-producing properties. From the medicinal point of view, they act through certain of their components on the tendency to sclerosis, in particular on that which affects the arteries. Hence they indirectly help to delay the ageing process in the 'nervous' type.

The Bilious Temperament

The dominant element characterising this type of Hippocratic temperament concerns the functions of the metabolism in breaking down the foods ingested (katabolism). This directly affects the liver which is the classic laboratory for this, as is its accessory, the gall bladder.

Typologically speaking, one can recognise the 'bilious' type by his dull, often even olive complexion. His face is triangular, his eyes lively and his expression domineering. His skin is dry and hot. His handshake, freely given, is frank and strong. He expresses himself forcefully and occasionally in a commanding tone. Uncompromising in his opinions, he cannot tolerate opposition and lives his life with a passion that must constantly fuel his pride. Having a tendency to distrust others, he is touchy about anything that concerns himself.

In the matter of health, the liverish nature of his

temperament predisposes the 'bilious' type to ailments affecting the digestive functions of that organ. It also affects the gall bladder. This leads initially to problems with indigestion and a tendency to constipation due to the slowing down of the flow of bile in the duodenum.

This survey of characteristics and behaviour patterns suggests that this type resembles the cosmic element FIRE. Its wine counterpart will be found in the Sauternes vintages. This region produces mellow and liqueur-like wines, whose topaz colour is not unlike bile—indeed they have been compared to 'a ray of sunlight concentrated in a glass'. This physical resemblance is even more striking in that, through their medicinal properties, the wines of Sauternes and Barsac exercise a physiological action on the gall bladder. Experience has proved that they promote the secretion of bile, and secondarily stimulate the liver functions. This link between FIRE and the LIVER did not escape the ancient Greeks. As we know, their legends include the myth of Prometheus, the son of the Titans, who had had the audacity to steal fire from heaven and was condemned by Jupiter to be chained to a rock where his liver was devoured by an eagle.

The Phlegmatic, or Lymphatic Temperament

Those belonging to this type of humour have recognisable physical and psychological traits. The dominant element is 'liquid', but the fluid is thick and stagnant in character, and is concentrated in the connective tissues. This physiological expression is linked with a slowing down in pituitary activity (the endocrine gland situated at the base of the skull) which controls the hormonal functioning of other glands governing internal secretion. This sluggishness in the biological processes causes oedemas, or swellings, in the internal areas.

Physically this type is thickset, with fat, flabby flesh, a

broad, hanging lower jaw, fleshy lips and a fat neck. The eyes lack vivacity. The handshake is limp and the skin surface feels damp and cold.

This physical heaviness is repeated in the psychological behaviour of the phlegmatic type. His movements are restricted and jerky, his speech hesitant and monotonous; his whole air is lethargic and has a certain apathy.

Because of this biological sluggishness, the phlegmatic type suffers from those symptoms that come under the heading of 'lymphatism', such as the existence of ganglions or swellings. He will also suffer from a lack of mineral salts, which predisposes him to rachitis (a softening of the bones). For the same reasons, metabolically he is likely to experience symptoms resulting from the retention of organic waste products—urates, oxalates, even urea.

These characteristic features link the 'phlegmatic' type with the cosmic element WATER, but in its stagnant form, needing help to be discharged. Its wine counterparts are the dry white wines, produced from vines planted beside water, whether rivers such as the Loire with its Muscadet and Sancerre or near the shores of lakes such as Lake Geneva, home of Crépy and Ripailles.

Apart from this 'humoral' resemblance, the above-mentioned vintages are rich in natural chemical compounds suitable for people of a phlegmatic temperament, especially alkaline carbonates which help to restore the balance of the system. They supply the mineral salts lacking in this type and, thanks to their diuretic properties, stimulate the excretory functions which are also lacking in efficiency.

A FINAL WORD

As I have indicated several times in this book, in discussing the virtues of the 'divine nectar' I have been writing under the aegis of Hippocrates, the Father of Traditional Medicine, and so my theme has been its medicinal properties.

In advocating this agreeable form of plant therapy, with its full flavours and wealth of health-giving ingredients, we have stressed the benefits that a natural product like wine can bring us whenever we feel ill or out of sorts. We have given several examples illustrating the healing effects of this beverage that gladdens men's hearts, delights the palates of connoisseurs but, most of all, will frequently supply the means to make good many physiological deficiencies affecting the main functions of the body. The reasons given for this have been backed by up-to-the-minute scientific research.

At a time when the health market is being flooded with synthetic products prescribed as healing agents, men and women, for their own protection and their own good, are turning more and more to natural medicines.

In this situation, the product of the vine holds a more than honourable place, so long as it is chosen to suit the individual's own temperament, responds to the existing health problem and, finally, is drunk wisely and in moderation. Our good master and colleague, François Rabelais, in perfect agreement with Hippocrates, could only give us his hearty approval.

GUIDE TO WINE THERAPY

Ailments	Recommended wines
Allergies	Corbières Côtes du Ventoux Minervois
Appetite (loss of)	Cahors Champagne (extra-dry) Clairette de Die Gaillac perlé Jurançon
Bacterial infections	Beaujolais Listrac Médoc St-Emilion
Cardiac problems	Champagne (extra-dry) Pouilly-Fuisse
Digestive ailments	Champagne (extra-dry)
Gastric problems	
Sluggish stomach	Médoc Monbazillac
Stomach pains	Barsac Sauternes
Intestinal problems	
Constipation	Anjou (sweet white) Bandol Bergerac Gaillac Vouvray (sweet white)

Ailments	Recommended wines
Diarrhoea	Médoc
Joint diseases	
Arthritis	Bandol
Osteoarthritis (onset)	Cassis
	Lirac
	Médoc
	Tavel
Osteoarthritis (chronic)	Corbières
	Côtes du Ventoux
	Minervois
Rheumatoid arthritis	Blancs de blanc
	Costières du Gard
	Crépy
	Sylvaner
Kidney problems	
Kidney stones	Crépy
	Ripaille
Urination	Muscadet
	Chablis
	Pouilly
	Sancerre
Metabolic problems	
Acidosis	Pouilly
	Sancerre
Cellulite	Gros Plan
	Muscadet
Convalescence	Champagne (extra-dry)
	Chinon
	Blanquette de Limoux
	Côte de Nuits
Detoxification	Champagne (extra-dry)

Ailments	Recommended wines
Diabetes	Bordeaux (red)
	Gaillac
	Riesling
	Sylvaner
Gout	Crépy
	Seyssel
Mineral deficiencies	Côtes de Bordeaux (premières)
	Champagne
	Chateauneuf du Pape
	Beaujolais
	Côtes du Rhône
	Sainte-Croix du Mont
	Saumur
Obesity	Beaujolais-Village
	Bordeaux (red)
	Gaillac
	Riesling
	Sylvaner
Uricaemia	Pouilly
	Sancerre
Vascular diseases	
Anaemia	Pomerol
Arteriosclerosis	Médoc
	St-Emilion
Hypertension	Champagne (extra-dry)
Myocardial infarction (heart attack)	Champagne (extra-dry)
	Blanc de blanc
Viral infections	Côtes de Bordeaux (premières)

MEDICAL WINE LIST

Alsace	Hypertension
Anjou (sweet)	Constipation
Bandol	Osteoarthritis
Barsac	Stomach pains
Beaujolais	Bacterial infections Mineral deficiencies
Blancs de blanc	Rheumatoid arthritis
Bordeaux (red)	Diabetes Obesity
Cassis	Osteoarthritis (mild)
Champagne (extra-dry)	Appetite (loss of) Convalescence Detoxification Digestive problems Hypertension Mineral deficiencies Myocardial infarction
Clairette de Die	Appetite (loss of)
Corbières	Allergies Osteoarthritis (chronic)
Côtes de Bordeaux (premières)	Influenza (prevention of) Mineral deficiencies
Côtes de Nuits	Convalescence

Côtes du Ventoux	Allergies Osteoarthritis (chronic)
Crépy	Gout Kidney stones Rheumatoid arthritis
Gros Plan	Cellulite
Listrac	Microbic infections
Lirac	Osteoarthritis (mild)
Médoc	Arteriosclerosis Bacterial infections Diarrhoea Rheumatism (acute) Sluggish stomach
Minervois	Allergies Osteoarthritis (chronic)
Muscadet	Cellulite Urination
Pouilly	Acidosis Uricaemia Urination
Ripaille	Kidney stones
Riesling	Diabetes Obesity
St-Emilion	Arteriosclerosis
St-Estèphe	Bacterial infections
Sancerre	Acidosis Uricaemia Urination

Seyssel	Gout
Sauternes	Stomach pains
Sylvaner	Obesity Rheumatoid arthritis
Tavel	Osteoarthritis (mild)
Vouvray	Constipation

APPENDIX
THE OTHER WINES OF EUROPE

As the scope of this book cannot extend to an exhaustive study of all the wines of Europe, only the best known wines will be given in each of the wine-growing countries concerned, comparing them to their French counterparts.

Country	Regional wines	French wines
Italy	Asti	Champagne
	Barolo	Côtes-du-Rhone
	Chianti (red)	
	Pasta wines	Beaujolais
	Red meat wines	Corbières
	Chianti (white)	Val-de-Loire
	Marsala	Banyuls
	Valpolicella	Médoc
Germany	Rheingau wines	Alsace-Sancerre
	Mittelrhein wines	Alsace-Sancerre
	Rheinhessen wines	Alsace-Sancerre
	Palatinate wines	
	reds	Anjou wines
	whites	Anjou wines
	Mosel wines	Alsace-Sancerre
	Rheinpfalz wines	Burgundy (red)
	Baden wines	Burgundy (red)
Switzerland	Valais wines	Burgundy (white)
	Pays de Vaud wines	Sancerre
	Dôle wines	Burgundy (red)
		Beaujolais
Spain	Malaga	Roussillon wines
	La Mancha	Roussillon wines
	Jerez	Roussillon wines
Portugal	Madeira	Roussillon wines
	Minho	Muscadet
	Dão	Burgundy (red)